Helen Lobato is an independent health researcher with a background in critical care nursing. She holds a Media Studies degree and was for many years a presenter of community radio programs focusing on women's currents affairs and women's health.

Gardasil
Fast-Tracked and Flawed

Helen Lobato

Published in Australia by Spinifex Press, 2017
Reprinted 2020

Spinifex Press Pty Ltd
PO Box 105
Mission Beach Qld 4852

www.spinifexpress.com.au
women@spinifexpress.com.au

Editors: Renate Klein & Pauline Hopkins
Cover design: Deb Snibson
Typesetting: Helen Christie
Typeset in Adobe Caslon Pro
Printed by McPherson's Printing Group

National Library of Australia Cataloguing-in-Publication data:
Lobato, Helen, author.
Gardasil: fast-tracked and flawed / Helen Lobato

9781742199931 (paperback)
9781742199948 (ebook : pdf)
9781742199962 (ebook : epub)
9781742199955 (ebook : kindle)

Includes bibilographical references
Gardasil (human papillomavirus vaccine)
Cervix uteri–Cancer–Vaccination–Complications–Australia.
Cervix uteri–Cancer–Vaccination–Australia.
Drugs–Side effects–Australia.
Cervix uteri–Cancer–Prevention–Australia

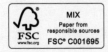

Contents

Acknowledgements

For over three decades, I have followed the issue of cervical cancer and I would like to take this opportunity to thank the many and growing list of activists who are vocal in their resistance to HPV vaccines. In particular I wish to thank Norma Erickson and Freda Birrell from SaneVax for their ongoing commitment to the truth and for their assistance in this project.

I also wish to acknowledge the young girls and now boys who have suffered ill health after vaccination with Gardasil and thank them for their courage in reporting their stories, many of which I have included in this book.

My sincere thanks go to my friends and family for their support while I have been engaged in writing this book.

To Renate Klein I extend my appreciation for all the help and support she has given me in this project, one we both truly believe in. As a biologist and a women's health researcher Renate's expertise has been invaluable.

And finally *Gardasil: Fast-Tracked and Flawed* owes its 'day in the sun' to Spinifex Press: Thank you to my wonderful publishers Renate Klein and Susan Hawthorne, to my editor and colleague Pauline Hopkins and office manager and friend Maralann Damiano. For Spinifex "publishing remains a political act."

Introduction

"Circumstantial evidence is a very tricky thing,"
answered Holmes thoughtfully. "It may seem
to point very straight to one thing, but if you
shift your point of view a little, you may find it
pointing in an equally uncompromising manner
to something entirely different ...
There is nothing more deceptive than an
obvious fact."

— Arthur Conan Doyle,
The Adventures of Sherlock Holmes
(1928, p. 208)

"Helen, I'm sorry to have to tell you but your smear test came back positive."

The phone call from my doctor was unexpected but my response was predictably anxious. Did I have cancer? Who will look after my family? Maybe it was a false positive result?

I was diagnosed with cervical dysplasia[1] in 1985. Since then I have closely followed the issue of cervical cancer and its recent resurrection from a disease of obscurity to one of new-found prominence.

---

1   When abnormal cells are found on the surface of the cervix, this is called dysplasia. Dysplasia may just go away on its own or, rarely, can progress to cancer. Another term for cervical dysplasia is cervical intraepithelial neoplasia (CIN) (Mayo Clinic 2016), see pp. 18–19 for more details.

After hearing that my Pap smear was abnormal I was very concerned that I might develop cancer. It may seem strange now but in those days we didn't talk about cancer in the open way that we do now; information was hard to find and there was no 'Dr Google' to turn to for 'advice'. The 1980s was also the decade when gay men began dying of a disease called acquired immune deficiency syndrome (AIDS). Sexual intercourse had become dangerous, one-night stands were problematic, and the use of condoms took on a whole new meaning. The media had a field day flashing pictures of dying men across our TV screens.

Health experts blamed these untimely deaths from AIDS on a new virus, the human immunodeficiency virus (HIV). Vast numbers of books were written and movies made on the topic, adding to the already feverish awareness and panic over this disease that, we were told, would cause more deaths than the black plague ever did.

It was also at this time that many scientists were suggesting that viruses might cause other types of cancer. The human papilloma virus (HPV) began to be talked about. Again the focus was on sexual activity and it was thought that a virus spread by sexual intercourse might be responsible for cervical cancer. HPV was assumed to be this virus.

The linking of cancer with sexual activity caused many women diagnosed with cervical dysplasia to feel very anxious. In *Cervical Cancer: A book for every woman*, Linda Dyson writes about her own experience (1996, pp. 86–87):

> In addition to coping with the fear of cancer, a woman who has just been told she has a cervical abnormality also feels threatened

4

at a social level … For some, the experience also led to the unhappy discovery that their partners had had other relationships.

According to Dyson, some women were indeed fearful of being seen as 'promiscuous' (pp. 84).

In a similar vein I began to wonder why I had developed dysplasia. How could I have gotten the HPV virus? This was before I knew that infection with HPV was very common and also, importantly, that it took more than the presence of this virus to develop cervical cancer.

But first things first: my immediate concern was to deal with my wayward cells. This process began with a referral to a gynaecologist who sent me off for a colposcopy, a procedure where my vulva, vagina and cervix were probed, scrutinised, scraped and sliced. This invasive technique has to be one of the most degrading and painful ever designed: I recall with horror being seated in a chair — not unlike a dentist chair — only it was my vagina that was opened up with a doctor peering in and probing me. I was assured that the procedure would not be painful but as he sunk his sharp blade into my cervix and cut out a tissue sample, I screamed and called him a liar. It hurt so very much!

The all-male medical team recommended a hysterectomy. Through their medical gaze they saw a 35-year-old woman and mother of three children who no longer needed her womb. They proposed to 'whip out my uterus'; for this very 'core' of me had presumably served its only purpose. Fortunately, I suspected this surgery to be problematic and am forever glad that I sought a second opinion on the necessity of a hysterectomy for cervical dysplasia, a disorder that was unlikely to have ever progressed to cancer. The overuse of hysterectomies for women's gynaecological ailments has always troubled me. There are around 30,000 hysterectomies performed in Australia annually with less than one per cent of these done for life-threatening reasons (Fox, 2015).

The story of cervical cancer and the development of vaccines against the human papilloma virus cannot be documented without looking at it within the context of the continued medical surveillance of women. The idea that the disease was associated with sexual intercourse had already become popular in the early years of the nineteenth century. Cervical cancer was purported to be common among poor city women but absent in nuns. Later it was found that religious sisters did also suffer the disease and that married women were frequently afflicted. How did the idea that this particular cancer involved promiscuous sexual activity ever arise? Was it because it was a cancer of a female reproductive organ that, according to the misogynist views of the times, existed for male sexual use first and foremost? Regrettably, even today, less newsworthy factors such as poor nutrition and the effects of environmental toxins along with hormonal disturbances, particularly among older women, are not given the same attention. It has been known for decades that glycogen[2] in the squamous mucosa of the cervix and vagina is depleted in cases of cervical cancer (Kent, 2012). But as we well know,

---

2   Glycogen is a stored form of glucose necessary for vaginal, vulva and cervical health. Vaginal lactobacilli use glycogen to produce lactic acid, which helps maintain low pH and dominance of lactobacilli and other acid-loving bacteria (Kent, 2012).

blaming sexual activities and producing a vaccine against a virus ensures vast profits for the pharmaceutical industry. Dealing with lifestyle issues does not.

The course and treatment of cervical dysplasia and cancer has changed dramatically since my experience. And new health policies are developed that will radically change the way that we detect cervical cancer such as the removal of the Pap smear test as the first line of defence (see pp. 28–29 for more on this questionable decision).

Fast-tracked and poorly-tested vaccines are now given to young girls and boys because of a link between the human papilloma virus and cervical cancer. As I will outline in detail, these vaccines are not only unproven but the vaccinated girls and boys can suffer devastating adverse effects that result in permanent ill-health and even death for some of them.

Following the story of the development and implementation of HPV vaccines is an uncomfortable ride. The rollout of the vaccines came after years of sensational media hype causing unnecessary fear and anxiety about a disease that began to decline in incidence in developed countries in the middle of the twentieth century.[3] In 2014, in Australia, 223 women died as a result of cervical cancer (Cancer Council Australia, 2016a). While every one of these deaths is of course tragic, there is no cervical cancer epidemic in Australia or in other developed nations. The disease is more likely to occur during a woman's middle years — between 35 and 55 years of age. Cervical cancer is rare in women under

---

3   From 1955 to 1992 the cases of cervical cancer and deaths fell by over 60% (National Institutes of Health, 2013).

the age of 20 years and approximately 20% of diagnoses are made in women older than 65 (National Cervical Cancer Coalition, 2016).

The story linking HPV to cervical cancer was substantiated in 1977. German virologist Harald zur Hausen claimed that HPV, known for causing warts, could also cause cervical cancer. Very soon he was joined by other men of science on a quest to verify zur Hausen's initial findings that linked HPV to a cancer which hitherto was thought to be connected to sexual promiscuity but also to poverty, nutritional deficiencies, habitual smoking and long-term contraceptive use.

Why and how the focus changed from an understanding of cervical cancer as a disease associated with social conditions and natural ageing to a cancer caused by a virus is part of this story along with the disastrous ramifications for the health of young girls and boys who, in the wake of a scare campaign, are now injected with HPV vaccines.

Chapter 1: Kristin Clulow

> I predict that Gardasil will become the greatest medical scandal of all times because at some point in time, the evidence will add up to prove that this vaccine, technical and scientific feat that it may be, has absolutely no effect on cervical cancer and that all the very many adverse effects which destroy lives and even kill, serve no other purpose than to generate profit for the manufacturers.
>
> — Bernard Dalbergue[4] *Health Impact News* (2014)

"It just breaks my heart," lamented Kristin Clulow.[5] In May 2008, the 26-year-old Australian woman received the first of the three shots of Gardasil, one of the human papilloma virus (HPV) vaccines on the market. Two weeks later, the fit young woman fell and broke her left foot and although perplexed at the ease at which she had incurred her fracture, she didn't think the two events were connected. In August 2008, she dutifully turned up

---

4   Dr Dalbergue is a former pharmaceutical industry physician with Gardasil manufacturer Merck (Health Impact News (2014).

5   Kristin Clulow's story is adapted, with permission, from my July 2013 interview, aired on 3CR Community Radio and found on my website <www.helenlobato.com>. It also contains information from a 2012 article; see Clulow, Kristin (2012).

at her doctor's office for her second shot of Gardasil. But shortly after this injection, Kristin's health began to unravel. It started with a temporary loss of vision and mobility problems that made it impossible for her to run, jump, dance or wear her beloved heels. Then her handwriting failed her: "Handwriting just doesn't suddenly go," she cried. Worse was to come when Kristin's speech became slurred: "They thought I'd had a stroke."

Her doctors insisted that these devastating symptoms were due to stress. They even had the nerve to claim she was making it all up! With the medical system unable or unwilling to help her, Kristin and her concerned parents went to see a neurologist. She was given the diagnosis of multiple sclerosis although tests did not confirm this. The prescribed treatment was methylprednisolone, commonly given to sufferers of this debilitating neurological disease. When the corticosteroid drug failed to relieve her symptoms, Kristin was referred to another neurologist. This specialist took one look at the sick young woman and straight away asked if she'd had any vaccines recently. When she told him she'd been given two shots of Gardasil, he replied "that will be it" for he'd recently treated 15 other girls with similar signs and symptoms.

One would have hoped at this point that this neurologist would have spoken out publicly against the vaccination program calling for caution. But instead all he could do for the sick woman was to give her more methylprednisolone after which Kristen continued to deteriorate and develop hallucinations and tremors — her right-sided weakness now extending to her left. This was in early 2009 and as Kristin recalls:

The next five months saw my health deteriorate further. I had blackouts, hallucinations, and struggled to do simple, everyday tasks. I couldn't sleep. I was constantly sick. I worked full time, attended physiotherapy, occupational therapy and speech therapy. When my symptoms extended to encompass my left side, my medical team went back to the drawing board (Clulow, 2012).

Finally, Kristin was given a positron emission tomography (PET) scan, a procedure similar to magnetic resonance imaging (MRI) that is able to show up the non-functioning parts of the body. In Kristin's case it was her cerebellum, the region of the brain that plays an important role in motor control. This vital part of her brain had ceased to function properly; she had severe damage to her nervous system and her immune system was so adversely affected that she succumbed to every infection going around.

The suggested treatment this time was immunoglobulin or human plasma prepared from the serum of between 1,000 and 15,000 donors per batch. Immunoglobulin is acquired from CSL Ltd which, interestingly, manufactures vaccines and is the Australian and New Zealand distributor of Gardasil.

Over the next 12 months Kristin received numerous treatments with intravenous immunoglobulin (IVIG):

I was in hospital every 28 days to receive intravenous immuno-globulin (IVIG) treatment. A great deal of this was sponsored by the Australian Red Cross, who I am forever grateful to. IVIG is the 'peacekeeper'. It is human auto-immune and helps to restore the body. The thing is it can only do so much. The rest is up to you. I underwent intense physiotherapy, occupational therapy, speech therapy and hydrotherapy (Clulow, 2012).

As to what was causing her suffering, Kristin was told that she had acute disseminated encephalomyelitis (ADEM), an immune-mediated inflammatory demyelinating condition that predominately affects the white matter of the brain and spinal cord (Brenton, 2016).

In February 2010, after almost two years of ill health, Kristin was able to return to Newcastle University where she began her Masters of Secondary Teaching Degree. Kristin continued working on returning her body to health with physiotherapy, gym work and of course the ongoing medical visits. And finally, in November 2011, she was given a repeat PET scan which showed her cerebellum "was coming back to life" (Clulow, 2012).

Kristin cares deeply about all the other girls who suffer ill health after Gardasil injections, and is furious that so many of them are not able to access the doctors, the diagnostic tests and the treatments they require. In her case, it had taken three years for her doctors to acknowledge that her symptoms had started after the Gardasil vaccinations and to treat her properly. "You need money and connections to get this help," a passionate but now very strong, young woman told me (Clulow, 2013).

Kristin has given an update on her progress in 'My Road to Recovery Post-Gardasil.' She writes that at a time when she "had reached a plateau", she heard from another 'Gardasil Girl' and found out that Melbourne homeopath Dr Isaac Golden who specialises in vaccination injuries was treating girls who had been adversely affected by Gardasil. According to Kristin: "His remedy does not reverse the effects of Gardasil. Instead, it helps the body in breaking down the barrier that Gardasil has created, allowing the body to recover itself" (2014). As a result of receiving this natural treatment, Kristin has noticed among other things an improvement in her mobility and a lessening of her tremors. A mineral analysis of her hair showed that her body was high in aluminium (2014). Aluminium is a neurotoxin. Aluminium compounds in a vaccine containing aluminium, added to boost immune function, can migrate and accumulate in the brain (Mercola, 2011). Each dose of Gardasil contains 225 micrograms of the neurotoxin.

In April 2007, Australia introduced the Gardasil vaccine for Australian girls aged 12–16 years. Gardasil is a vaccine purported to act against four strains of HPV, two of which are said to be associated with the development of cervical cancer. Yet there are more than 100 strains of HPV and it is well known that around 80% of people acquire the virus at some point in their lives. It is also a fact that most of these infections clear up naturally and that in about 90% of cases this happens within 2 years (World Health Organisation, WHO, 2016b).

SaneVax, the website of an international group of concerned individuals (some of them whom lost their daughters after Gardasil injections), provides information and awareness about vaccination practices. They report that there have been over 50,000 adverse events from vaccination with HPV vaccines including 315 deaths (SaneVax, Inc. 2017b). However, these statistics are far from accurate. According to the U.S. National Vaccine Information Center (2017b) it is estimated that only 1% to10% of adverse vaccine reactions are ever reported. Unfortunately we are looking at much higher figures of injured girls and boys.

As noted above, developed nations such as Australia do not have high levels of cervical cancer. Since the National Cervical Screening Program began in 1991, the number of deaths from the disease have halved (Australian Institute of Health and Welfare, AIHW, 2012–2013). Nevertheless, in 2007, the Australian Government added HPV vaccines to its immunisation program with the result that children who are most unlikely to develop cervical cancer within the period that the vaccine remains active in their bodies which is said to be about 5 years, are injected with these drugs. It is not currently known if booster shots will be needed (The *Dijene* HPV Test, 2017). Other nations are to be congratulated for questioning their HPV vaccination programs. On June 14, 2013, the Japanese Health Ministry issued a nationwide notice that the so-called 'cervical cancer' vaccinations should not be recommended for girls aged 12 to 16 (The Asahi Shimbun, 2013). This precautionary move followed reports of 1,968 cases of possible adverse effects including body pain, numbness and paralysis. Anna Fifield, writing for the *Washington Post*, reports that Japan is finding it difficult to resume its recommendation for the vaccines. She quotes Miyako Hagiwara whose daughter became ill after she was vaccinated in 2013. "I forever regret having my daughter get her vaccination. I wish I could suffer for her," she said (Fifield, 2015). The Japanese government is undertaking an investigation into the HPV vaccines with a view to decide whether it will continue its current stance or resume recommendation for vaccination (Paras, 2016).

Unlike Japan, Australian health authorities have not taken any action to ensure the safety of its young girls. Not only has

Australia failed to take similar action, in 2013, the government-subsidised vaccination program was extended to 12- and 13-year-old boys, supposedly to provide protection against genital warts and cancers of the penis and rectum, and to reduce transmission of HPV to girls. At the very least like Japan, Australia should cease its promotion of HPV vaccines and warn young people of adverse effects that may arise if they agree to be vaccinated with Gardasil. We really need to know why medical practitioners such as the neurologist who recognised Kristin's symptoms as related to Gardasil have not spoken publicly about what is happening to girls (and now boys) who have been injected with HPV vaccines. Such doctors are obviously aware of the extreme side effects and yet appear reluctant to speak out. Australian health professionals and the public are able to report an adverse event occurring after the use of a particular drug on the Database of Adverse Event Notifications[6] found on the Therapeutic Goods Administration (TGA) website.

Although our mainstream media remains silent about the problems emanating from this vaccination program, some doctors are reporting the adverse effects on young women's health. In the *BMJ* (British Medical Journal) *Case Reports* authors Deidre Little and Harvey Rodrick Grenville Ward of Australia reported the case of a patient with amenorrhoea who had noticed that her usual regular menstrual cycle had changed, becoming irregular and then scant after her HPV vaccinations (Little and Ward, 2012). The authors explain that it is very rare for the condition

---

6   Database of Adverse Event Notifications <https://www.tga.gov.au/about-daen-medicines>

known as premature ovarian failure to occur at such an early age and that the annual incidence is 10 per 100,000 between 15 and 29 years of age. Premature ovarian failure is a serious health event for young girls and one that adversely affects their ability to have children (Little and Ward, 2012).

We can hope that there are many more conscientious medical practitioners and researchers who go on to report their findings on the problematic nature of this vaccine.

This story of Gardasil will probe the reasons for the introduction of the HPV vaccine. Many questions come to mind but an important one is how and why this vaccine program was implemented when deaths from cervical cancer in Australia and other industrialised nations were already in steep decline, thanks to regular Pap smears, and improvements in general health, nutrition and sexual hygiene.

Chapter 2: Cervical Cancer

> There were persistent rumours in the presidential palace that Juan Perón could not stand the odours emanating from his wife's dying body. Some of his aides reported that he entered her room very rarely and when he did he kept a muslin mask over his face, like a bee keeper.
>
> — Llana Löwy, *A Woman's Disease: The history of cervical cancer* (2011, p. 20)

In 1949, the 30-year-old wife of Juan Perón, the President of Argentina, was diagnosed with cervical cancer. Eva, the actress and passionate political activist had little patience for illness and ignored the constant pain and bleeding along with the advice from her doctors. But denial can only last so long and soon the malignancy spread to her ovary at which point there was little hope of survival.

As a nurse I have cared for women with advanced cervical cancer, an awful terminal disease. Often it is a gradual decline towards death accompanied by the indignity and nuisance of foul vaginal discharge. Measures such as frequent baths and the topical use of aromatherapy help to mask unpleasant odours and provide a necessary distraction from the failing body, the once strong self.

While stories about breast cancer victims are plentiful, it is rare to read the tangible accounts of women with cervical cancer, particularly stories of older women with the disease. This is surprising when, according to researchers at Keele University in the UK 20% of cases of cervical cancer and almost half of the deaths occur in women aged over 64 (*The Guardian*, 2015).

Eileen, who had a family history of cancer, was diagnosed at 64 years of age with cervical and uterine cancer after experiencing episodes of heavy bleeding. The mother of three's treatment consisted of radiation and chemotherapy followed by a total hysterectomy and oophorectomy (removal of the ovaries). She is now cancer-free and urges other women to avail themselves of preventative testing (Centers for Disease Control, CDC 2014).

Cervical cancer is a malignant tumour arising from cells of the cervix — the lower, narrow section of the uterus — that have undergone changes, first causing a pre-cancerous condition called cervical dysplasia. Cervical dysplasia is usually symptomless with the condition picked up when a woman has a Pap smear (WebMD, 2017). While it is not cancer, it is referred to as a pre-cancerous condition (Macmillan, 2015). Most cases of dysplasia, also known as cervical intraepithelial neoplasia (CIN), do not progress to cancer. There are three stages of CIN indicating the severity of the disease. CIN 1 is mild dysplasia and may go away on its own without treatment. It may be judicious to have follow up smears just in case. The second stage of dysplasia is known as CIN 2 or moderate dysplasia. The third stage is CIN 3 and classified as severe dysplasia. CIN 2 and 3 are usually treated by removing the abnormal cells (Macmillan, 2015).

The stage from the development of abnormal cervical cells to the development of cervical cancer can take years and may depend on the health of the particular woman (Dyson, 1986, pp. 13–16). Linda Dyson, author of *Cervical Cancer: A book for every woman*, suggests that the manner or speed at which the disease progresses may be influenced by factors such as a woman's "immunity to disease, or other factors such as whether she smokes or uses an oral contraceptive" (1986, p. 16).

There are two types of cervical cancer. Squamous cell carcinoma is the most common cervical cancer and accounts for over 70% of cervical cancers. A less prevalent form of the disease, adenocarcinoma, arises in the glandular cells and is more difficult to diagnose than squamous cell cancer. The risk factors for cervical cancer are many and include smoking, a weakened immune system, multiple pregnancies, a family history of the disease, the prolonged use of birth control pills and, more recently, HPV, the human papilloma virus (Cancer Council Victoria, 2015a). The daughters of women who took diethylstilbestrol (DES)[7] while pregnant — commonly called DES daughters — have around a 40 times higher risk of developing clear cell adenocarcinoma[8] of the cervix than women who did not take DES. This equates to around 1 in 1,000 DES daughters who

---

7   DES is a hormonal drug that was prescribed to women to prevent miscarriage between 1940 and 1971. It had serious consequences for both mothers taking it and their offspring resulting in an increased risk of miscarriages, ectopic pregnancies and stillbirths. DES women have more than twice the risk of an early menopause (National Cancer Institute, NCI 2011).

8   Clear cell carcinomas make up 4% of adenocarcinomas and are associated with DES daughters (Perunovic, 2013).

develop this form of cervical cancer (National Institutes of Health, 2011).

In the nineteenth century, 80% of all cancer fatalities in women were from breast or uterine cancer, with cancer of the uterus being responsible for most of these deaths (Löwy, 2011, p. 29). Prior to the development of surgery, belladonna, hemlock, strychnine, lead and even mercury were applied to the lesions in the hope that they would rid the body of the "cancerous poison" (p. 31). Once surgery became available, treatments such as cauterization were used to address horrific complications which can occur in advanced cervical cancer; one of these was the formation of a fistula, a hole "between the vagina and urethra and/or rectum" (pp. 40–43). Such an unfortunate condition was accompanied by incontinence. For these affected women there was loss of "blood, urine and faeces" accompanied by despair. Understandably they experienced their ill health as "a fate worse than death" (pp. 41–42). Today the most common treatment for cervical cancer is surgery and/or a combination of chemotherapy and radiotherapy (Cancer Council Victoria, 2015b). These days most women who are diagnosed early with cervical cancer or cancer in situ can be effectively treated and cured. In Australia the five-year survival rate is 72% (Cancer Council Australia, 2016a).

Numerous theories as to the cause(s) of cervical cancer have come and gone over the decades. There are the early nineteenth-century physicians who claimed that 'sexual excesses and immorality' were involved, for it was observed that the disease was found in larger numbers among poorer, city women than amongst married and financially more secure women living in rural areas (Löwy, 2011, p. 140). Domenico Rigoni-Stern, an Italian surgeon, followed this dubious line of reasoning and claimed that cervical cancer rarely occurred in nuns (p. 140). This theory was later discounted when a study revealed that in fact religious sisters were subject to the disease too, and that, contrary to prevailing opinion, women in long-term relationships also developed cervical cancer. Further research by British physician J.C.W. Lever found that "single women bear a proportion of 5.83 per cent, married women 86.6 per cent, and widows 7.5 per cent," of cases of cancer of the womb (p. 141).

With the notion that sexual excesses and/or immorality were the cause of the disease discredited, researchers began to suspect that a "chronic irritation" or an underlying inflammatory process could be the missing link. In the case of cancer of the uterus it was proposed that the trauma of childbirth itself could be a risk factor. Such speculation might explain why there was more cervical cancer among women of low socioeconomic status than among women of means. Poorer women tended to have more children, lived harsher lives and possibly received less medical care, as well as missing out on much-needed rest and recovery time after the birth of their children (Löwy, 2011, p. 143).

I believe these early researchers were on the right track when they proposed that social circumstances such as poverty and inequality were in some way implicated in the disease process. British psychologist, author and researcher Susan Quilliam documented these lifestyle factors that might increase the chance of becoming ill with cervical cancer in her 1989 book *Positive*

Smear. Written just before the idea that the human papilloma virus might be involved, she stressed the importance of a balanced diet and claimed that deficiencies in vitamin C, beta carotene and folic acid were common in women with cervical pre-cancerous cells. Quilliam strongly emphasised the importance of a healthy environment, good hygiene and excellent nutrition as prerequisites for good health and resistance to disease (1989, pp. 96–98). When discussing the causes of cervical cancer, she doesn't shy away from a conversation about the contraceptive pill and how it has a negative effect on natural immunity as well as a propensity to lessen the body's ability to use folic acid (p. 99).

Regrettably, since Quilliam's 1989 book, the pendulum has swung back to regarding cervical cancer as a disease associated with sexual activity. HPV is now seen as the main culprit and any discussion that there may be other factors that lead to this disease is silenced in the mainstream media.

Why, when and how this has happened is crucial to the story of *Gardasil: Fast-Tracked and Flawed*.

Chapter 3: Pap Smears

> Women are driven through the health
> system like sheep through a dip.
>
> — Germaine Greer, *The Whole Woman*
> (1999, p. 109)

Affordable access to a smear test has long been regarded as a woman's right. Along with the advent of second wave feminism came a timely rise of activism around women's health issues. One of the many health provisions fought for and won was cervical smear testing for women. Many Western countries established and implemented national education and screening programs. Women were urged to submit themselves to a Pap smear — a rather uncomfortable and invasive test — to detect changes in the cells of the cervix which may, if left unobserved and untreated, lead to cervical cancer.

In 1914, George Papanicolaou began working at Cornell University Medical College's Department of Anatomy. It was while studying the sex cycle of guinea pigs that he discovered how to perform cytological examinations of vaginal smears. In 1920, he began to practice his newly acquired skill, obtaining smear samples from his wife (poor Mary), and abnormal smears from ill female patients at the Cornell Clinic who on further physical examination were found to have cervical cancer. Although this incidental discovery led to the auspicious development of the Pap smear, a cheap and relatively easy-to-perform test for pre-cancerous and cancerous conditions, it was not introduced into general (and still only limited) use until the 1940s (Shepard, 2011).

It would take another decade or so for governments to begin introducing cervical cancer screening. The UK government did so in 1966 and found the demand very low because many women lacked confidence in the screening test (Löwy, 2011, p. 129). British health authorities, concerned that the women at greatest risk were not consenting to smear testing, developed an educational campaign promoting the benefits of the procedure. This community health promotion included the production and showing of educational films containing the very clear message that it was a woman's duty to have the test, if only because her family needed her. An example of the persuasive intent is evident in one of the film titles: "Stay young, stay with us" (Löwy, 2011, p. 133).

Although there is government and public support for cervical cancer screening throughout the world, many countries lack well-funded, organised programs such as exist in the UK, Australia and other developed nations. From the 1960s to 1991, cervical cancer screening was available to women in Australia on an opportunistic basis in that the test was done on the request of the doctor or the woman herself. Then, in 1991, an organised program was set up which in 1995 became the National Cervical Screening Program. Such organised programs are more effective than those of an opportunistic nature because they specify a defined target population and include policies on method and interval of screening. Europe has few such organised programs with many countries relying on opportunistic screening. Screening in the USA and Canada varies from opportunistic to organised screening, and among the Latin American countries, Chile and Colombia boast national organised programs that have been operating for at least 15 years. Of all the countries in Africa, only South Africa has an official national cervical screening policy. Cervical cancer is the second most prevalent cancer among women there, with the highest incidence among black women between the ages of 66 to 69. In 2014 South Africa began vaccinating school girls against HPV. Developing nations such as India have no organised screening program, with testing only available to a small population of mainly urban women (International Agency for Research on Cancer, IARC, pp. 119–140, 2005).

In Australia, it is standard practice for doctors to remind their female patients to keep their Pap smears up to date. However, few women would be aware that cervical cancer is not responsible for huge numbers of deaths in developed countries including Australia. Furthermore, the Pap smear test itself is not without problems or critics, with many feminists declaring it part of an interventionist model of care. As Germaine Greer said in her book, *The Whole Woman* (1999), "… screening is many times more likely to destroy a woman's peace of mind than it is to save her life" (p. 115).

This important point is echoed by British general practitioner Jane Chomet and co-author Julian Chomet. Dr Jane Chomet became interested in cervical cancer after Dr Papanicolaou visited the Royal Free Hospital where she was studying medicine in the early 1960s. Her son Julian, a medical journalist, joined her in writing *Cervical Cancer: All You and Your Partner Need to Know about Its Prevention, Detection and Treatment.* The authors claim that concern about the impending tests and treatments, along with the extreme trepidation that they may indeed have cancer, are common among women (1989, pp. 124–127). This was my experience when I was diagnosed with cervical dysplasia. Moreover, I suspect that the harsh treatment I was given was not warranted.

When considering the benefits of cervical screening it needs to be stressed that for every life saved, masses of women have to undergo screening and many of them subsequently are treated for conditions which would not have led to cancer. Abnormal smear tests lead to unnecessary interventions such as occurred over a five-year period in Bristol when 15,000 smears were said to be abnormal and more than 5,500 women were given additional testing that resulted in treatment (in Greer, 1999, p. 111). Not only were these women likely to be subjected to colposcopies (see: Introduction p. 5), cone biopsies,[9] diathermy[10] and cryosurgery,[11] they would also have unnecessarily worried about cancer and their future reproductive health.

---

9   A cone biopsy involves removing the abnormal cervical tissue and a cone of tissue underneath it. It can be done for CIN, carcinoma in situ and micro-invasive cancer (Dyson, 1986, p. 70).

10 Diathermy is used to burn the abnormal area of the epithelium and is performed under anaesthetic (Dyson, 1986, p. 69).

11 Cryosurgery is done for minor abnormalities, mostly CIN 1 or 2. It does not need an anaesthetic. Cryosurgery is a freezing technique applied to the

Since the Australian National Cervical Screening Program began in 1991, the number of deaths from the disease have halved (Cancer Council Australia, 2017). But, as Germaine Greer points out in *The Whole Woman*, deaths from cervical cancer had already fallen before the introduction of organised screening programs (1999, p. 109). Although opportunistic screening played a large part in the overall decline, I wonder if the success may also be due to improvements in living conditions and the overall better health of women during the latter half of the twentieth century in Western nations.

The following poem reflects one woman's concerns about the increasing medicalisation of women (1989, p. 108):

> I am, a lady with infections
> Bladder kidney vaginal yeast
> I am a beast
> PMS wench sore back and headache
> Cysts on ovaries tubes uterus cervix
> Breast cancer scare
> Pap smear fear
> — Anonymous poem, *Anarcha-feminist hag mag* No. 4

If it appears that I am overly critical of Pap smear tests which I have no doubt saved many women's lives, it is because I believe that more attention needs to be paid to preventative measures such as the correction of dietary deficiencies, cessation of smoking, use of condoms and the promotion of drug-free methods of birth control. Also, there must be changes to the socioeconomic

---

affected area which results in blistering and the abnormal cells are therefore removed (Dyson, 1986, p. 68).

conditions of disadvantage and the effect these factors have on women's general health and wellbeing. For example, Aboriginal and Torres Strait Islander women have poorer health compared to non-Indigenous women, leading to a lower life expectancy.

It is also interesting to note that countries such as France which did not have a national Pap smear screening program until 2003 was found in 2006 to have tumour rates on a par with other nations that had previously established screening programs (Löwy, 2011, p. 139).

But despite the problems associated with Pap smears, I strongly believe the diagnostic smear test needs to be retained. Clearly women are still developing dysplasia that can lead to the development of cervical cancer. The earlier the disease is diagnosed, the sooner treatment can be commenced.

For these reasons it is extremely concerning that the Australian government has announced that from December 1, 2017 an HPV test will replace the current Pap smear test. From December 1, the age at which women are advised to start cervical screening will be raised to 25 years from the current 18 years. The interval between tests will be increased to five years from the existing two-year interval (Department of Health, 2015). The sample is obtained in the same way that a Pap smear is taken in that cervical cells are collected and examined.

The new HPV test is predicated on the theory that HPV causes cervical cancer. However, it is not a test for cervical cancer as such but a test for the presence of the human papilloma virus. HPV is a very common virus — so much so that most of the adult population has been infected at some point in their life with the virus. If the new test finds that a woman has HPV type 16 or 18, she will be given a colposcopy to look for any pre-cancerous cervical lesions. And if the HPV test finds any of the other high risk strains of HPV, then a Pap test will be ordered to ascertain if a colposcopy is required (Sifferlin, 2014). All of this of course means that the new HPV test will most likely result in more colposcopies, and a lot of unnecessary worry for women who return a positive HPV test.

Of particular concern are the women who test negative for HPV but who may still have cervical cancer. HPV-negative cervical cancers are present in many types of cervical cancers. Zhao MD and his colleagues report that large-scale studies reveal the existence of HPV-negative cervical cancers present in almost all types of cervical cancers (Zhao MD *et al.*, 2014). According to Bosch *et al.* (2002), there has been little investigation of older women with cervical cancer, but it is likely that the HPV-negative cancers can be found in this group of women. These HPV-negative women will not have their disease found as early as they would have with a routine Pap smear. In other words, many early cases of *possible* cervical cancer will be missed. Any change to Australia's successful screening program needs to consider the case of DES daughters who are at risk of clear cell adenocarcinoma of the cervix, a less common form of cervical cancer which "develops from the mucus-producing gland cells of the endocervix … the part of the cervix closest to the body of the uterus" (American Cancer Society, 2017). Adenocarcinoma is more difficult to diagnose because it originates higher in the cervix and annual Pap smears and a colposcopic examination of both the cervix and the vagina are recommended (DES Action, 2016). These changes to the screening guidelines are highly problematic. Will they result in more women seeking HPV vaccination (those women who are not already HPV-positive)?

In sum, although the diagnostic Pap smear test is not perfect, in countries which have national cervical screening programs there has been a significant and consistent decline in cervical cancer and resulting deaths. In Australia, there was a 50% reduction in new cases and deaths from cervical cancer from 1991 (the year in which the national screening program began) to 2002, after which time results have plateaued (Australian Institute of Health and Welfare, AIHW, 2016). In countries without organised screening programs, the rate of cervical cancer ranges from 50 to 90 per 100,000 women whereas in Western nations which encourage regular screening, cervical cancer incidence is 5 to 8 per 100,000 women (Heitmann and Harper, 2012).

For all these reasons, Pap smears should remain the front line diagnostic tools given their proven success. HPV was only proposed as the cause of cervical cancer in the late 1980s and many disagreed about the validity of this now entrenched theory. Using a 'preventative' HPV test and then possibly the HPV vaccine if the woman has no HPV infection to replace a proven diagnostic tool — the Pap smear — poses serious health risks for many women.

In the following chapter I will shed light on the development of the questionable HPV thesis as the cause of cervical cancer.

Chapter 4: The Human Papilloma Virus

> We all have been taught to greatly fear viruses
> — and yet scientists are now discovering that
> they are fundamental parts of life, made by
> the millions by all healthy cells.
>
> — Dr Roberto A. Giraldo, physician and specialist
> in internal medicine, infectious and tropical diseases
> (in Roberts, 2008)

The disease in which cells start to grow out of control and eventually cause death to the organism owes its name 'cancer' to Hippocrates. The Greek physician had noted the way tumours spread out, reach into, and invade neighbouring body parts, resembling "finger-like spreading projections" which "called to mind the shape of a crab" (Mandal, 2014).

Professor Karol Sikora, in an article published in the *Daily Mail*, explains how we used to talk about cancer (Sikora, 2009):

> In the beautiful film Shadowlands, about the life and love of writer C. S. Lewis, there's a memorable scene where his fiancée Joy Gresham, the American poet, is found to have breast cancer. No mention of the disease is ever made. But you can almost smell the disinfectant in the hospital. The starched nurses' uniforms with their austere hats would put you off asking too many questions

Since the 1960s, there has been a vast improvement in our understanding of cancer and in the way we treat and interact with those who suffer this disease. The hospital of the 1960s was a closed place with interaction between staff and patients taking place in hushed, serious tones. Mother's Day fundraisers for breast- or other types of cancer were not in existence, nor were social media platforms telling us all about celebrities fearful of developing breast cancer and undergoing double mastectomies rather then taking the risk.[12] In the general community and in doctors' rooms, cancer was referred to as the 'Big C'. Doctors and nurses ducked the word; they told patients they had a lump, a cyst or a growth. Today in Australia, there is no avoiding the truth as cancer is named a leading cause of death with 1 in 2 Australian men and women predicted to be diagnosed with some form of cancer by age 85 (Cancer Council Australia, 2017a).

Whereas infectious diseases such as influenza, pneumonia, diarrhoea and tuberculosis were among the leading causes of death in the early 1900s, by the 1950s, many of these diseases were in decline. This improvement was mainly due to welcome changes in living conditions like access to potable water, sanitation, and better nutrition. But just as the rate of infectious diseases was declining, death from cancer rose (Australian Institute of Health and Welfare AIHW, 2005), along with the level of fear about the disease. The public wanted answers, they wanted to know the cause. Most of all they wanted a cure.

---

12 In May 2013, Angelina Jolie underwent a preventative double mastectomy after tests showed that she carries the BRCA1 cancer gene (Jolie Pitt, 2015). Women who have a fault in the BRCA1 or BRCA2 gene have an estimated 30–60% risk of breast cancer (Cancer Australia, 2017c). It is important to note that Jolie might never have gone on to develop cancer, for not every woman with this gene mutation will get breast or ovarian cancer (Cancer Australia, 2017c).

Perhaps part of the reason for the increase in the rate of cancer was that people were living long enough to develop the disease. Nevertheless, as the nature of cancer was puzzling, in the early twentieth century, microbiologists began to look for cancer-causing germs. A connection between organisms such as bacteria or fungi and cancer could not be established, but that was not the end of the matter. The task of finding the cause of cancer shifted to virologists who, aided by increasingly sophisticated technologies, took up the cudgel — this time searching for hypothetical cancer-causing viruses.

As the work intensified, it became clear that there was a real problem with the very idea that viruses cause cancer. For while cancer isn't contagious — that is, we don't catch cancer from family members or friends by breathing the same air or touching each other — viruses are contagious and can be passed from one person to another. Cancer causes cells to increase and grow rapidly and out of control, whereas viruses kill cells. When a virus enters a living cell, it uses the cell's resources to reproduce. In the process, the cell dies. Despite this clear difference between the behaviour of viruses and cancer, the hunt for cancer viruses continued with virologists becoming prominent and influential players in the cancer industry (Duesberg, 1996, pp. 89–91).[13]

---

13 In this chapter I have referred to the work of Professor Peter Duesberg who became a controversial figure after he questioned whether the human immunodeficiency virus (HIV) caused AIDS. In 1992, Duesberg and Jody Schwartz, both molecular biologists at the University of California at Berkeley, announced their concern over the 'HPV-causes-cervical-cancer' theory, claiming that there was a lack of consistent HPV DNA sequences and consistent HPV gene expression in tumors that were

I often wonder about the ability of the scientific community to have most of the world believing that viruses, and not lifestyle and environmental changes, are the cause of these horrid cancers. But then breakthroughs in science are good news stories and enthusiastically told by the media. Ian Harris is the author of *Surgery, The Ultimate Placebo* (2016). Although his subject is surgery and not viruses and vaccines, his work provides food for thought on why there is this pervasive public acceptance of scientific and medical 'wisdom'. In this book, Harris writes that the benefits of many forms of surgery are overstated and that the risks are greater than we are led to believe. He says that the public are kept in the dark about the failure of many common surgical operations to make any difference to the patient.

In his chapter 'The science of medicine — or lack of it' he touches on the misrepresentation of scientific facts by the media. He also points out that the more advanced the science, the more the media reports it. The reason that the media makes such a fuss of seemingly good health stories, he says, is because the public love science and welcome success stories that help people (Harris, 2016, pp. 56–57).

Following on from Harris' observations, it is easy to see how public fear about cancer combined with good news about the latest scientific breakthroughs has led to billions of dollars spent on cancer research. In December 1971, after the American

---

HPV-positive. They suggested that rare spontaneous or chemically-induced chromosome abnormalities might be the culprits, meaning that carcinogens could be the primary inducers of abnormal cell proliferation rather than a virus such as HPV (Duesberg and Schwartz, 1992).

people had made it abundantly clear they wanted a cure for cancer, the second-leading cause of death in the United States, President Nixon signed the National Cancer Act (Dana-Faber Cancer Institute, 2013). Forty-five years later, the mystery of cancer remains. Nixon's 'War on Cancer' falsely raised the hopes of Americans (and the world) and despite billions of dollars, the rates of cancer continue to escalate (Cuomo, 2012).

Alas, Nixon's war against cancer — which was in fact a war against nature — was illusionary. In this story about cervical cancer and current treatments it may be helpful to understand the disease as proposed by Michael Coleman from the Cancer Research UK Cancer Survival Group in his essay 'War on cancer and the influence of the medical-industrial complex', published in the *Journal of Cancer Policy* (Coleman, 2013). He describes cancer as "a uniquely diverse constellation of diseases that stem from spontaneous or induced errors in the complex genetic systems that have evolved over millions of years to regulate the reproduction of our own cells" (p. 33).

He also tackles the use of the 'metaphor of war' (p. 31):

> *Waging war* against a disease that is so intrinsic to our cellular biology is even more quixotic than declaring a war on terror, drugs or religion. *War* is more than just a metaphor. It distorts political thinking about cancer with the illusory clarity of victory and defeat.

Given the confused logic and contradictions in the virus-causes-cancer story, it is reassuring to read the enlightening work of the late investigative journalist and author Janine Roberts. In *Fear of the Invisible: How Scared Should We Be of Viruses and Vaccines, HIV and Aids* (2008), Roberts suggested that rather than seeing viruses as harmful we need to see them for what they are: part of life. As she put it: "… we make them, shape them and live within a sea of them" (p. 58). Roberts further claimed that viruses are made out to be enemies that must be attacked in order for pharmaceutical companies to be the beneficiaries of a multi-billion dollar 'war on terror' (p. 58).

Unfortunately, most of us have not had access to Janine Roberts' important work and so we obediently swallow the words of mainstream media reporting the latest science 'breakthroughs'. Certainly, those involved in the search for a virus that causes cervical cancer were encouraged by the resurfacing belief in the 1960s and 1970s that sexual activity was involved in the transmission of cervical cancer (as espoused by nineteenth century Italian surgeon Domenico Rigoni-Stern, see p. 21).

In the late 1960s, it was postulated that the herpes simplex virus (HSV) was the cause of cervical cancer until it was found that 85% of American adults had been infected with this virus without getting cervical cancer and that many women who had cervical cancer had never been infected with the herpes virus. Not about to give up on the idea that the herpes virus caused cervical cancer, researchers pressed on and proposed a "hit-and run hypothesis that the herpes virus briefly infects cervix cells … and makes some mysterious, undetectable change" (Duesberg, 1996, p. 110). Then it supposedly disappears with the cancer developing many years later.

Common sense eventually prevailed but not until the early 1990s, when this rather spurious idea was abandoned (Duesberg, 1996, p. 110). Meanwhile, another virus was receiving equal scrutiny and raising hopes. In 1977, Harald zur Hausen had begun exploring the idea that the human papilloma virus could be the cause of cervical cancer. In the early 1980s, the German virologist found the human papilloma virus, HPV type 16, in approximately 50% of cervical tumours and HPV type 18 in approximately 20% of cervical tumours (Smith, 2014). Initially, when zur Hausen approached some pharmaceutical companies with his idea of developing a vaccine against HPV, he was turned down. They told him it wouldn't be worth their while developing a vaccine and felt there were more pressing problems to work on (McIntyre, 2005).

But overall, the scientific community welcomed the news of a cancer-causing virus even though other institutions such as the International Agency for Research on Cancer (IARC) were wary and stated: "Although evidence for an association between cervical cancer and sexual activity has been available for over a century, the causal role of a sexually transmitted infectious agent has not yet been proven" (IARC, 1989).

Despite this lack of consensus, in 1989, Professor Ian Frazer and Dr Jian Zhou from the University of Queensland in Australia received funding from CSL Ltd, formerly known as the Commonwealth Serum Laboratories to begin work on a vaccine which "would prevent carcinogenic changes believed to result from HPV infections" (Wilyman, 2015, p. 345).

Scottish-born Ian Frazer had moved to the University of Queensland in 1985 where he began working on papilloma virus immunology and a vaccine. But developing the vaccine was not straightforward for "HPV proved impossible to grow in the lab"

(University of Queensland, 2017). "Most viruses can be grown in the lab because the cell lines that are grown are 'permissive', which means that when a virus gets inside, all the machinery necessary for that cell to make lots of copies of the virus is present," explains Madonna King, author of *Ian Frazer: The Man Who Saved a Million Lives* (King, 2013 p. 84). "HPV is different," writes King (p. 84). Undaunted by the challenge, Ian Frazer and the late Jian Zhou, an expert in gene technology, 'reasoned' that "If HPV couldn't be grown … then perhaps they could build their own version of the virus" (University of Queensland, 2017).

Investigative journalist and author Janine Roberts comments on this inability of scientists to produce the HPV virus from cell cultures. "So far scientists have failed to persuade any cell culture to produce this virus, even cultures made of cervical cancer cells." Roberts quotes the International Agency for Research on Cancer (IARC) which reports that HPV "cannot be propagated in tissue culture" (IARC, 1995) and so the virus is "produced by cloning" meaning "made in a laboratory"(Roberts, 2009, p. 1):

> … these vaccines are the product of a new synthetic vaccine industry based, not on isolating viruses, but on reproducing short lengths of genetic codes postulated to come from proteins that once formed the outer coat of the virus (Roberts, 2009, p. 1).

Roberts explains that sensitive new testing enables the study of small fragments of genetic code found in cellular material. These fragments of code are said to have come from the outer coating of HPV and it is on the manufactured versions of these proteins that the vaccine is based. These are known as virus-like particles (VLP).

She goes on to explain how Gardasil is made using these virus-like particles:

… these are put into cells and multiplied in yeast cell cultures, or in baculovirus cultures for Cervarix. Fluid from the culture containing these particles is then used as the vaccine. The vaccines are thus certain to contain many particles from the yeast fungi or baculovirus, and whatever additives are used — and thus Gardasil is not officially recommended to those who are sensitive to yeast (Roberts, 2009, p. 1).

Madonna King describes the moment when Frazer and Zhou looked at the photographs of their creation, the virus-like particle: "They had so often imagined this moment, now it was difficult to fully comprehend. Here in front of them was a HPV VLP in black and white" (King, 2013, pp. 88–89). What the two scientists had developed was "the shell of a virus without the infectious DNA inside it". It was "a history-making moment: the creation of HPV-like particles using DNA recombination technology" (p. 88).

The race was on: they now needed a patent and they needed a commercial partner. The accolades continued with the awarding of the 2008 Nobel Prize in Medicine to Harald zur Hausen for discovering that HPV causes cervical cancer (Nobel Prize, 2008). But, as Janine Roberts has stated: Harald zur Hausen "failed to find a way to persuade cells to make his virus" (Roberts, 2008, p. 1).

However, over the years, the theory that HPV causes cervical cancer has become thoroughly entrenched. As a result, whenever cervical cancer is discussed in the media, it is bluntly stated that this cancer is caused by the HPV virus. And the popular narrative then continues by stating that we now have HPV vaccines that will prevent the development of this cancer.

Unfortunately, thousands of young girls who follow this advice, are now suffering severe adverse reactions after HPV vaccinations. Tragically the stories of these sick girls permeate the pages of *Gardasil: Fast-Tracked and Flawed.*

Jasmine is a writer and co-founder of Brisbane's first domestic violence memorial. Jas followed her doctor's advice and had her Gardasil shots. Here is her story:

> If I'd known at the age of 22 that Gardasil would destroy almost three years of my life, I never would have gone through with it. I really knew nothing about it, other than what my doctor told me — which was that it was a great new vaccine, and that I should definitely get it 'while the Government was offering it for free.' I wasn't told anything about the serious side effects and young women who had been admitted to hospital with serious muscular issues — or worse, had died.
>
> Following my first injection I experienced almost immediate 'crawling' sensations on my legs, which at the time, I figured was just a lack of magnesium. It wasn't too bad, and the discomfort mostly went away; however, after the second injection it came back — tenfold. As a result, I had three years of chronic muscular/nerve pain (at times it was a dull ache, at others, it felt like fire ants stinging me all over my body) that impacted everything from my relationship (due to the depression and insomnia that I developed) to my ability to study and enjoy life. I also became addicted to taking Panadol and Nurofen every single night for those following years, as it was the only thing that helped.

At no time did any doctor appear even remotely interested in discussing the correlation between when my pain had started, and the Gardasil injections. Instead I was told that I probably just had fibromyalgia (I didn't). I was lucky enough to be told about a registered GP in Sydney who offered holistic treatments, and in 2009 travelled six hours to her centre to try and find answers. She was the only one who made the link.

In 2010, after several years of naturopathic treatment and continuing pain, I eventually recovered. I remember seeing my original doctor around that time and when I told her what I had been through, all she said was, "well it's a good thing you had the injections, at least you won't get HPV now."

To this day I'm still disgusted that I was never offered any information on the side effects, let alone given options to report my injury (I still never have, as it was years before I knew it was even an option), and I believe this particular vaccine needs to be pulled from production. To know that so many women have gone through worse than what I have is completely unacceptable. I've decided to speak out now because I don't want any further women and girls harmed by Gardasil (Jasmine, 2017).

Chapter 5: HPV Vaccines

> Vaccination policies in Australia need to be
> scrutinised because the use of a medical
> intervention in the prevention of infectious
> disease has serious health and social
> implications.
>
> — Judy Wilyman, 'A critical analysis of the Australian
> government's rationale for its vaccination policy'
> (Wilyman, 2015, p. iv)

There are many concerns about the wholesale adoption of HPV vaccines and one of these is the nature of the vaccine itself. The World Health Organisation (WHO) describes a vaccine as:

> … a biological preparation that improves immunity to a particular disease. A vaccine typically contains an agent that resembles a disease-causing microorganism, and is often made from weakened or killed forms of the microbe, its toxins or one of its surface proteins. The agent stimulates the body's immune system to recognize the agent as foreign, destroy it, and 'remember' it, so that the immune system can more easily recognize and destroy any of these microorganisms that it later encounters (WHO, 2016a)

Well and good — or is it?

Not according to vaccine researcher Dr Lucija Tomljenovic who discusses the way vaccines act in the human body in a letter titled 'Forced Vaccinations: For the Greater Good'. This letter was delivered to the Californian State Senate Committee in

2015 when a mandatory vaccination law was being debated (Tomljenovic, 2015).[14]

Tomljenovic describes how vaccines fail to bring about cellular immunity and thus protection from disease (Tomljenovic, p. 7, 2015):

> … vaccines primarily stimulate humoral immunity (antibody-based or Th2 responses) while they have little or no effect on cellular immunity (cytotoxic T-cells, Th1 responses), which is absolutely crucial for protection against viral as well as some bacterial pathogens.

Tomljenovic suggests that this failure to bring about cellular immunity may be why booster shots of vaccines are often needed (p. 7). Vaccination immunity doesn't last, whereas natural immunity continues over time. There are two parts to the immune system. One is the humoral immune system which primarily produces antibodies in the blood in response to the presence of foreign antigens in the body. This is where vaccines have most influence. Then there's the cellular or cell-mediated system of immunity that rids the body of foreign antigens, and in the process manifests as an acute inflammatory response of the body exhibiting signs such as fever and malaise. If a vaccine stimulated the whole immune system the vaccinated person would have an inflammatory response and get all the symptoms of disease (Incao, 2006).

Philip F. Incao MD sums it up like this (2006):

---

14 SB 277 is a Californian law which requires mandatory vaccination as per schedule for all school children (California Legislative Information, 2015).

Vaccinations are usually effective in preventing an individual from manifesting a particular illness, but they do not improve the overall strength or health of the individual nor of the immune system.

But immunity is rarely described in this way and so vaccines are largely accepted as the way for communities to stay healthy and stem the spread of disease.

Currently, there are three HPV vaccines on the market: The quadrivalent HPV vaccine GARDASIL® was produced to be protective against four HPV types: 6, 11, 16, and 18. The bivalent vaccine CERVARIX® to be protective against two HPV types: 16 and 18, and GARDASIL®9 to be protective against nine HPV types: 6, 11, 16, 18, 31, 33, 45, 52, and 58.

HPV vaccines are sold as preventatives against cervical cancer, whereas in reality they are vaccines which are protective against a few strains of the human papilloma virus. This vaccination program began and continues in spite of the fact that cervical cancer is a rare outcome of a persistent infection with one or more cancer-causing types of human papillomavirus (AIHW, 2015). The plain fact is that 90% of HPV infections are asymptomatic and naturally cleared by the immune system within two years (WHO, 2007).

In 'The causal relation between human papillomavirus and cervical cancer', Bosch *et al.* state that the HPV has been proposed as the first ever identified, 'necessary cause' of a human cancer and that "cervical cancer does not and will not develop in the absence of the persistent presence of HPV DNA." (Bosch *et al.*, 2002). However, in the same paper the authors state that studies have "unequivocally shown that HPV DNA can be detected in adequate specimens of cervical cancer in 90–100% of cases." This contradicts their previous statement that the disease won't occur without the presence of HPV. That it will not develop without the presence of HPV DNA is untrue for according to the Centers for Disease Control and Prevention (CDC), only 91% of cases of cervical cancer are found to be HPV positive. In the USA over the period of one year, there were 11,771 cases of which only 10,700 were HPV positive (CDC, 2016). Bosch *et al.* supported the decision to trial the vaccines in spite of the fact that the evidence supporting causation had not been found. Although they state that the "proof of cause was elusive," they argued that trials of a vaccine should continue, claiming that "all scientific work is incomplete" (Bosch *et al.*, 2002). In her 2015 PhD thesis 'A critical analysis of the Australian government's rationale for its vaccination policy', Judy Wilyman states that this is a case where these scientists saw it as "their duty to trial an HPV vaccine even though their evidence that HPV 16/18 were the determining cause of cervical cancer was incomplete" (Wilyman 2015, p. 224).

There are further problems with the claim that HPV vaccines are effective against cervical cancer. HPV vaccines have never been tested against cervical cancer outcomes. It can take decades from HPV infection to the development of cervical cancer so such definitive testing is simply not possible (WHO, 2009).

Instead, a surrogate endpoint was used to support the conclusion that HPV vaccines would be effective in preventing cervical cancer. Surrogate endpoints or markers are used when the use of real clinical outcomes as endpoints is impractical.

For example, clinical trials may take too long to determine outcomes, they may cause discomfort or harm to persons involved, or they may just be too expensive to undertake (Chin, 2016). Chin states: "in many instances surrogate endpoints have turned out not to be predictive of clinical response at all." But, according to Manhattan-based Dr Kelly Brogan, the use of a surrogate "is considered acceptable because we can't otherwise prove a non-event is attributable to an intervention" (Brogan, 2015). However, the surrogate endpoint chosen to support the hypothesis that HPV vaccines may be effective against cervical cancer was not appropriate as we shall see.

The suitable surrogate end-point (or marker) chosen for the efficacy of the HPV vaccine was cervical intra-epithelial neoplasia (CIN) grade 2/3 lesions, and adenocarcinoma in situ (WHO, 2007). This surrogate end-point was decided even though these precursor lesions are common in young women under 25 years and rarely progress to cancer (WHO, 2008, p. 8). In fact, only 5% of HPV infections go on to become CIN grade 2 or 3 lesions within three years. Of those CIN 3 lesions that don't clear up naturally, only 20% turn into an invasive carcinoma within five years and 40% go on and develop into invasive carcinoma in 40 years (Heitmann and Harper, 2012).

In sum, very few of these CIN 2 and 3 precursor lesions in young women develop into cancer so it is difficult to support their use as end-points or markers for cervical cancer.

This is an incredible situation and I invite all readers to pause for a moment and reflect on what this means. All over the world millions of girls continue to be injected with a vaccine which has only been measured against a surrogate endpoint — precursor lesions — that most often do not lead to cervical cancer. If the vaccine had no adverse effects, we could just rail against the capitalist nature of Big Pharma, but in the light of the thousands of girls (and boys) who fall seriously ill after HPV shots, we have to also seriously question the ethics inherent in the HPV vaccine industry and ask why governments continue to subsidise them.

But clearly Merck takes a different view. In her 2015 PhD thesis, Judy Wilyman researched the HPV trials. She found that when it was revealed that women (15 to 26 years old) who were given the vaccine developed fewer precursor lesions (grade 2/3) than women who were not given the vaccine, Merck claimed that the vaccine prevented "100% of high-grade disease and 'non-invasive' cervical cancers associated with HPV infection" (p. 241). But in reality, Wilyman contends, this result depended on the group studied and that the significant reduction in precursor lesions was only observed in the study group that had not been infected with HPV 16/18 at baseline (FDA Merck Ltd 2006, in Wilyman 2015, p. 241). It is important to note that if CIN 3 does change into invasive cancer this progression occurs over 8.1 to 12.6 years. However, the longest follow-up study for the phase three clinical trials examining the efficacy against precursor lesions was only four years. "Therefore, the correct assumption is that precursor lesions in this age-group are not an indication that cervical cancer will develop from high-risk HPV infections" (p. 241). In other words, Wilyman contends, "there is no evidence of how much cervical cancer this vaccine may prevent" (p. 242).

Contrary to what the medical fraternity and the vaccine manufacturers would have us believe, to this day, none of the HPV vaccines have ever been proven to prevent a single case of cervical cancer. Diane Harper, one of Merck's HPV vaccine researchers, and now a whistleblower, has admitted that vaccinating young girls will not to protect them against cervical cancer for it can take a decade or more for dysplasia to develop. As Harper put it:

> It is silly to mandate vaccination of 11- to 12-year-old girls. There also is not enough evidence gathered on side effects to know that safety is not an issue. This vaccine has not been tested in little girls for efficacy. At 11, these girls don't get cervical cancer — they won't know for 25 years if they will get cervical cancer (in Sharav, 2013).

"Merck knows this," Harper continued. "To mandate now is simply to Merck's benefit, and only to Merck's benefit" (in Sharav, 2013). This point has been supported by health researcher Renate Klein: "Let's not forget that Gardasil was fast tracked through the FDA, a process normally reserved for life saving drugs" (Klein, 2008).

Luckily, for Merck, as Klein observes, Gardasil has given the pharmaceutical company necessary funds to pay compensation owed to the victims of Vioxx, the arthritis drug which caused thousands of heart attacks and deaths. Also in receipt of proceeds from this vaccine is the Commonwealth Serum Laboratories (CSL), the Australian and New Zealand distributor of Gardasil which receives royalties from Merck (in Klein, 2008).

For a drug or vaccine to be fast-tracked it must be a treatment for a serious disease and it must fill an unmet medical need. Did Gardasil fulfill this unmet need? Not according to Norma

Erickson, one of the founders of the SaneVax organisation who agrees that while cervical cancer is a serious disease, Gardasil does not fulfill an unmet need:

> Due to regular cancer screening and appropriate medical follow-up when abnormal cervical cells are detected, cervical cancer rates in the United States have dropped over 74% and continue to decline. This is the case in most developed countries around the world. So, where is the 'unmet medical need?' (Erickson, 2010).

In spite of the fact that there was no 'unmet' need, as cervical cancer rates had fallen over the past few decades at least in developed countries as a result of cervical smear testing and improvements in the standard of living, HPV vaccines continue to be injected into young people. The year 2016 was the tenth anniversary of the first HPV vaccination Gardasil in the USA. In Australia, vaccination was started in April 2007 (Colvin, 2007).

Gardasil is a genetically engineered vaccine. Similar to the situation with genetically engineered foods, we do not know enough about the long-term heath effects of such experimental products on the bodies of developing adolescents.

Passionate health reformer and author, Joseph Mercola, asks:

> What happens when foreign DNA is inserted into the human body is a mystery. Will it trigger undesirable changes in human cells or tissues? Will it combine or exchange genetic material with human DNA? Will it transfer to future generations? No one knows … (Mercola, 2012).

While the answers to these questions remain unknown, what we do know is that there have been thousands of reports of adverse reactions following the administration of HPV vaccines.

These adverse reactions manifest as:

> sudden collapse with unconsciousness within 24 hours seizures; muscle pain and weakness; disabling fatigue; Guillain-Barré Syndrome (GBS); facial paralysis; brain inflammation; rheumatoid arthritis; lupus; blood clots; optic neuritis; multiple sclerosis; strokes; heart and other serious health problems, including death, following receipt of Gardasil vaccine; (Fisher, 2016).

A study of the contents of the Gardasil vaccine reveals that along with the proteins of the human papilloma virus types 6, 11, 16, 18, it contains many additives including aluminum, yeast protein, sodium chloride, L-histidine, polysorbate 80, sodium borate, and water for injection (Merck, 2011).

Of particular concern is the presence of sodium borate, which is the main ingredient in boric acid, often used to kill cockroaches (Off The Radar, 2016). Sodium borate and another ingredient, polysorbate 80, have been linked to infertility. Indeed, concern over this additive has resulted in borax-containing products imported into the European Union required to carry the warning 'May damage fertility' and 'May damage the unborn child' (Off The Radar, 2016). We should not be surprised then that in January 2016, the American College of Pediatricians found it necessary to issue a press release warning that Gardasil could be "associated with the very rare but serious condition of premature ovarian failure" (Field, 2016). The American College of Pediatricians expressed concern that the vaccine's effect on long-term ovarian function had not been studied. They state that since Gardasil was licensed in 2006, there have been over 200 reports made on the Vaccine Adverse Events Reporting

System (VAERS) involving amenorrhea, premature ovarian failure (POF) or premature menopause, 88% of which have been associated with Gardasil, and Cervarix being responsible for the other 12% (American College of Pediatricians, 2016).

Gardasil includes significant amounts of aluminium used as an adjuvant[15] to increase the body's immune response. It beggars belief that this heavy metal is allowed to be put in vaccines when studies have shown that aluminum adjuvants can result in the metal entering the brain (National Vaccine Information Center NVIC, 2006). The presence of aluminium can cause nerve cell death as well as inflammation at the injection site leading to chronic joint and muscle pain. This is extremely important because Gardasil contains 225 micrograms of aluminium (CSL, 2016). This is bad enough, but gets worse when one realises that the recommended course of Gardasil is three shots bringing the total of the aluminium injected to 675 mcg. Even more incredible is the information that Merck's latest HPV vaccine Gardasil 9 — contains even more aluminium. One dose of Gardasil 9, approved by the FDA in 2014 for the prevention of cervical, vulvar, vaginal and anal cancers contains 500mcg: more than twice as much aluminum as the original Gardasil vaccine (Erickson, 2014c). This is even more alarming when one reads that Merck recommends two or three shots of Gardasil 9 depending on the age of the recipient in which case the total amount of aluminium injected ranges from 1,000 to 1,500 mcg (Merck, 2016).

---

15 A substance that is added to a vaccine to increase the body's immune response to the vaccine (Centers for Disease Control and Prevention (CDC, 2015.)

Regrettably there is no reason to think that Cervarix, the vaccine designed to prevent infection from HPV types 16 and 18, is any safer. GlaxoSmithKline's vaccine has been used in Europe and Australia since 2007. Although Cervarix was licensed in the USA in 2009, the manufacturer GlaxoSmithKline has since ceased production due to low demand (Mulcahy, 2016).

Cervarix, the bivalent HPV vaccine includes a new adjuvant system called ASO4 which contains aluminium hydroxide and another immune modulator called MPL which is monophosphoryl lipid A. This causes a much stronger immune response (GlaxoSmithKline, 2007). Cervarix was studied for less than six years and in fewer than 1200 healthy girls under the age of 15. It was not tested against a true placebo but was compared against the hepatitis A vaccine and other childhood vaccines that can also cause adverse reactions (National Vaccine Information Center, NVIC, 2016). Is it any wonder that the number of girls and boys suffering adverse effects after HPV vaccines continues to rise?

It is not difficult to see why HPV vaccines are associated with more deaths, and serious adverse effects than other vaccines. Alton reports that: "The HPV vaccine is linked to a higher risk of disability and premature death" (Alton, 2015). In 2008, the National Vaccine Information Center in the USA published a Gardasil risk report which found that death and serious adverse events are reported three to 30 times more often after vaccination with Gardasil than after the meningococcal (Menactra) vaccination (Fisher, 2009b).

So where is the outrage over the inclusion of dangerous additives in these now common HPV vaccines? Have health authorities responded to the concerns expressed by The American College of Pediatricians? Do people not realise that these toxic chemicals are injected into human adolescent bodies? We really have to ask the question: how do HPV vaccine manufacturers get away with it?

Jana, from Nove Zamky, Slovakia, tells the story of her two daughters, now 21 and 23 years of age, who, on recommendation from their gynaecologist, were vaccinated with Cervarix in 2009. Jana regrets giving her consent and says that she has caused her daughters' medical problems by allowing them to be injected with this HPV vaccine. One of her daughters started experiencing ticks on her face which she did not have before. She also started coughing for no apparent reason. All the tests that were conducted came back normal. It has been more than six years and these problems have not stopped. Her second daughter stopped having menstrual periods some time after the vaccinations. After numerous tests it was confirmed that her daughter's ovaries have stopped producing eggs and she is now infertile (Jana, 2016).

Malinda (USA) tells her daughter's story.

My daughter, Jessica had the Gardasil vaccinations between August 2006 and April 2007. She had her first one before she left for college. Shortly thereafter, she started calling us and telling us that she was losing a lot of hair. Next came the stomach-aches. Soon, she had such bad stomach-aches. Soon came issues with constipation. We had gone to a few doctors that tried her on Irritable Bowel Syndrome medicine and probiotics for stomach acid. Nothing seemed to make a difference.

Over the next two years her symptoms progressively got worse. Also, in the meantime we went from one doctor to the next. We even went to Mayo Clinic in Rochester, MN. Their final diagnosis was Chronic Fatigue Syndrome and Fibromyalgia. Why? What caused this to a girl that used to be perfectly normal, healthy, athletic and super bright?

Her symptoms have progressed to extreme fatigue, swollen lymph nodes, inflammation, achy muscles, sores in her nose, bladder infections, yeast infections, abnormal pap smear, insomnia, heart palpitations, foggy concentration, headaches, extreme stomach bloating and stomach pains, horrendous menstrual cycles, and an overall ill feeling. Never really feels good. Some days are worse than others. Jessica can get a good night's sleep and then feel like she has a hangover in the morning.

Some of the issues I am concerned about with her is did Gardasil push her body into menopause? Will Gardasil cause her cervical cancer? Will Gardasil cause her to have infertility issues? Did Gardasil push her body into an autoimmune disorder which causes this overall general ill feeling she has?

We are currently using food supplements and vitamins to try to make her feel better. It seems like she may have a better day and then boom, the next day is not so good (Green, 2009).

"It went too fast, it went too fast without any breaks," said the aforementioned Merck ex-researcher Diane Harper who had devoted nearly two decades of her career to research on HPV. According to Dr Harper,

> … the vaccine has not been out long enough for us to have post marketing surveillance to really understand what all the potential side effects are going to be. We feel it is very safe [but] we don't

know yet what's going to happen when millions of doses of the vaccine have been given and to put in process a place that says you must have this vaccine, it means you must be part of a big public experiment. So we can't do that until we have more data (in Fisher, 2008).

Dr Deirdre Little (see page 15–16) is a general practitioner in the small town of Bellingen, in New South Wales, Australia. Little comes face to face with girls and young women who visit her practice feeling ill after the Gardasil vaccination. She is a rare breed of doctor for she is speaking publicly about the HPV vaccination program. She relates the story of a 16-year-old female patient who suffered premature menopause after her Gardasil vaccination. Unfortunately, this is not an isolated event for other Gardasil vaccinated girls have reported to her that their periods are scanty and irregular. On further research she discovered that according to the Australian Therapeutic Goods Administration (TGA), the Gardasil manufacturer did not conduct studies on Gardasil and ovarian function, or any studies regarding ongoing effects on fertility. Little explains how the vaccine was fast-tracked, adding that when there is an urgent need for a vaccine it is fast-tracked. However she added that of these fast-tracked vaccines "one in three to one in five are withdrawn from the market because of adverse reactions." Dr Little wonders why HPV vaccines were introduced at all when Pap smear programs had already reduced cervical cancer by 70 percent. She also comments that there are no studies showing how much cancer an HPV vaccine can prevent (Family Life International, FLI, 2013).

This is Dr Little's advice to parents of young girls: "I personally do not think there is enough information in the government handouts for any parent to give a valid informed consent regarding Gardasil" (FLI, 2013).

Chapter 6: Investigate before you vaccinate

> Informed consent prior to any medical
> intervention is a basic human right.
> By definition, informed consent gives you
> the right to analyze the risks and benefits
> of the proposed medical intervention then
> refuse (opt out) of having the procedure
> performed if the risks outweigh the benefits
> for you as an individual. The problem is
> many people seem to have forgotten
> vaccines are a medical intervention.
>
> — Norma Erickson,
> 'Vaccines: The Battle for Informed Consent'
> (Erickson, 2015)

It takes courage to speak out about the widespread practice of vaccination which is sold to the general public as indispensable. In Australia, the number of vaccines given to young children continues to increase and by the time a child goes to school s/he will have been given 41 vaccines, or even 46 if s/he also had the recommended influenza shots (Dorey, 2016). The Australian National Vaccination Program also includes HPV vaccines for all girls and boys aged 12–13 years. The course of Gardasil consists of three injections given over six months.

According to the Australian Immunisation Handbook, the minimum intervals for HPV vaccination is one month between doses one and two; and three months between doses two and three (Department of Health, 2015).

One important reason for the overall public acceptance of the practice of vaccination is our neglect of history in regard to disease and prevention.

Although many scientists attribute the decline in infectious diseases to medical interventions such as vaccination, opposing voices have argued that it was *political, social and economic interventions in behaviour and the environment* and not the use of drugs and vaccines that precipitated the welcome change. One such notable dissenter was the Austrian philosopher and author Ivan Illich who wrote:

> The combined death rate from scarlet fever, diphtheria, whooping cough and measles among children up to fifteen shows that nearly 90 percent of the total decline in mortality between 1860 and 1965 had occurred before the introduction of antibiotics and widespread immunization. In part, this recession may be attributed to improved housing and to a decrease in the virulence of micro-organisms, but by far the most important factor was a higher host-resistance due to better nutrition (Illich, 1976, p. 16).

The practice of vaccination has its origins in a scientific model of health which minimises the importance of social, political and ecological factors in the development of disease. Cervical cancer is a case in point. Over the past few decades the rate of incidence has notably decreased in developed nations where the standard of living is high. Also, organised screening programs are in existence. According to Parkin and colleagues in their work on global cancer statistics, cervical cancer now accounts for only

3.6% of new cases of cancer in developed nations (Parkin *et al.*, 2005, p. 91).

Sadly these figures are not replicated in the developing world where cancer of the cervix makes up 15% of new cancers (Parkin *et al.* 2005, p. 91). That there has been such a welcome reduction in cases of this cancer in developed countries such as Australia is largely due to our standard of living that includes access to affordable health care, availability of nutritious food and quality education. For an example of how social and political factors impinge on women's health we only have to look at Indigenous Australia as Indigenous women have twice the risk of developing cervical cancer (Australian Institute of Health and Welfare, AIHW, 2012–13 p. 25). Shockingly, their mortality rate is four to five times higher than that of non-Indigenous women (AIHW, 2012–13, p. 30).

Improving socio-economic conditions such as decent health care, education and access to quality food takes time, involves politics and is not as newsworthy or lucrative as marketing a new vaccine and extending its reach. In 2012, the then Federal Health Minister, Tanya Plibersek, launched the world's first national human papilloma virus (HPV) immunisation program for boys aged 12–13, which began in February 2013 (Cancer Council Australia, 2013). It is astounding that an extension of this problematic vaccination program to include boys was given the go-ahead when there had already been serious safety issues associated with the Gardasil vaccination program for girls. By 2013, when the program to vaccinate boys was commencing, Australia's database of adverse event notifications (DAEN) had

1,961 reports of adverse events occurring in girls following the cervical cancer vaccination (TGA, 2017). These figures would be much higher if there was a requirement for mandatory reporting of adverse events. If this were the case, the government would take lodged adverse effects seriously and the media would report them. But expanding the market by finding new consumers makes more money for the vaccine industry which is what the Gardasil vaccination program for boys has achieved.

Unsurprisingly we are now told that boys too get sick after HPV vaccinations (and some have died). On June 19, 2013, Joel Gomez, a healthy 14-year-old boy had his first dose of Gardasil. Joel did not report any adverse reactions following this first vaccination to his family or his physician. Then two months later he was given a second injection of Gardasil after which he went home and went to sleep. He was found unresponsive in his bed the following morning (Lee, 2015).

An autopsy was performed on August 23, 2013 by James K. Ribe, MD, senior deputy medical examiner of Los Angeles, California revealing the following findings:

> … a long narrow band of dark reddish discoloration which is somewhat darker than the rest of the myocardium, extends over a length of 6 cm and has a width of 0.4 cm extending from the anterior base of the heart almost to the apex … this lesion is limited to the anterior free wall. Both lungs are extremely heavy. The lung parenchyma is dark-purple-red and completely soaked with edema fluid and blood (Lee, 2015).

The following is the conclusion that senior cancer pathologist Dr Sin Hang Lee gave in his expert report in the Matter of Gomez v. United States Department of Health:

> In the opinion of this author, there is sufficient evidence based on which to conclude that the vaccine Gardasil® is capable of causing sudden unexpected death in certain predisposed vaccinees that Gardasil® did cause or contributed to a myocardial infarction in the decedent, and that the second dose of Gardasil® finally caused a fatal hypotension in this case on the day of vaccination. There was no other plausible cause for the death of Joel Gomez at the night of August 19, 2013 (Lee, 2015).

Dr Lee explains the role Gardasil could have played in the death of this healthy 14-year-old boy:

> After he was given the first dose of Gardasil® vaccine on June 19, 2013, Joel Gomez, a football player, apparently developed a silent localized myocardial infarction during one of these cytokine[16] surges probably when he was playing football at a time as the demand for blood perfusion to the heart muscle was high. A sudden reduction of blood perfusion apparently caused a transient ischemia and an infarction in the left ventricle where the demand of oxygen is most critical in competitive sports. But Joel did not have any significant clinical symptoms during and after the infarction. The lesion began to heal.
>
> However, after the second Gardasil® vaccination a new surge of cytokines directed more myocardial depressants to the heart,

---

16 Cytokines are small proteins that are secreted by certain cells of the immune system. They play a part in bodily processes such as inflammation and immunity. Different cytokines are responsible for symptoms that accompany infection, inflammation and pain (Gillaspy, 2017).

causing an episode of hypotension when Joel went home in the evening of August 19, 2013. The heart with a damaged left ventricle now under the effects of a new wave of myocardial depressants could not pump enough blood into the arterial circulation to maintain the needed blood pressure.

Joel came home and went to bed when his blood pressure was dropping. The patient eventually died of left heart failure due to insufficient blood perfusion to the heart muscle and brain (Lee, 2015).

The US Food and Drug Administration (FDA) had licensed Gardasil, quadrivalent HPV vaccine, for use in males 9–16 years of age for the prevention of genital warts caused by HPV types 6 and 11 in October 2009. A search of the US Government's VAERS, The Vaccine Adverse Event Reporting System, reveals that there have been 5,127 reports of adverse effects in males who have been given HPV vaccines by September 2016. The adverse effects included anaphylaxis, peripheral neuropathy, Guillain-Barré syndrome, syncope, heart arrhythmias and convulsions (NVIC, 2017).

It would be safe to say that these serious side effects and deaths in both girls and boys following HPV vaccination come as no surprise to Canadian researchers Lucija Tomljenovic and Christopher A. Shaw who report that there have been numerous studies and case reports documenting neurological and autoimmune adverse reactions (ADRs) following the use of various vaccines. The most frequently reported reactions manifest as arthritis, vasculitis, systemic lupus erythematosus (SLE), encephalopathy, neuropathy, seizure disorders and autoimmune demyelinating disease syndromes. In their 2012 research article 'Death after Quadrivalent Human Papillomavirus (HPV) Vaccination: Causal or Coincidental' they discuss how they developed a protocol based on an analysis of cases of sudden death following vaccination with the quadrivalent HPV vaccine (also called qHPV vaccine) or Gardasil. The purpose of the protocol is to determine whether the serious autoimmune and neurological symptoms following HPV vaccination were causal or merely coincidental. Their paper includes a discussion of the deaths of two young women:

Case 1

A 19-year-old female without a relevant medical history and taking no drugs expired in her sleep, approximately 6 months after her third and final qHPV vaccine booster and following exacerbation of initial vaccination-related symptoms. She had last been seen alive by her parents the previous evening. Her symptoms started after the first qHPV injection when she developed warts on her hand that persisted throughout the vaccination period. In addition, she suffered from unexplained fatigue, muscle weakness, tachycardia, chest pain, tingling in extremities, irritability, mental confusion and periods of amnesia (memory lapses). The autopsy was unremarkable and failed to determine the exact cause of death. Internal examination revealed some minor changes involving the gallbladder and the uterine cervix (both of which on further examination by microbiological studies and histology revealed no significant disease). After a full autopsy no major abnormality was found anatomically, microbiologically or toxicologically that might have been regarded as a potential cause of death. Histological analysis of the brain hippocampus, cerebellum and watershed cortex allegedly revealed no evidence of neuronal loss or neuroinflammatory changes. However, the autopsy report did not specify which immune antibodies and stains were used for histological investigations (Tomljenovic and Shaw, 2012 p. 2).

Case 2

A 14-year-old female with a previous history of migraines and oral contraceptive use who developed more severe migraines, speech problems, dizziness, weakness, inability to walk, depressed consciousness, confusion, amnesia and vomiting 14 days after receiving her first qHPV vaccine injection. These symptoms gradually resolved. However, 15 days after her second qHPV vaccine booster she was found unconscious in her bathtub by her mother 30 minutes after she had entered the bathroom to have a shower. Emergency help was summoned and arrived quickly. Resuscitation efforts were attempted. The paramedic noted that the patient was found without a pulse. Upon arrival at the hospital and approximately 30 minutes later, the patient suffered cardiac arrest. Resuscitation was terminated approximately 40 minutes later and the patient was pronounced dead (Tomljenovic and Shaw, 2012 p. 2).

Tomljenovic and Shaw examined brain tissue from the two women who tragically died after vaccination with Gardasil. Their tests revealed an autoimmune vasculitis (inflammation of blood vessels) brought on by the cross-reactive HPV-16L1 antibodies binding to the wall of blood vessels. The researchers claim that their finding of HPV-16L1 particles in cerebral blood vessels and adhering to the walls of these vessels clearly shows that "vaccine-derived immune complexes are capable of penetrating the blood-brain barrier" (p. 3).

The HPV quadrivalent recombinant vaccine Gardasil is a mixture of virus-like particles derived from the L1 capsid proteins of HPV types 6, 11, 16 and 18. These virus-like particles are absorbed by way of amorphous aluminium hydroxyphosphate sulfate adjuvant. Cerebral vasculitis results in inflammatory destruction of blood vessel walls causing haemorrhage and ischaemia (restricted blood flow) to surrounding tissues. And as we know, a large number of the complaints reported to VAERS following HPV vaccination are clearly suggestive of cerebral vasculitis manifesting as migraines, syncope, seizures, tremors and tingling, myalgia, locomotor abnormalities, psychotic symptoms and cognitive deficits. These findings are of extreme concern to Tomljenovic and Shaw who claim that HPV vaccines containing HPV-16L1 VLPs (including Gardasil and Cervarix) are unsafe for some people. Alarmingly, it is unknown which individuals are prone to an adverse reaction after HPV vaccination (Tomljenovic and Shaw, 2012 p. 9). And yet the vaccinations continue unabated.

Nicole Alexandra, from Sacramento in California wrote about her experiences in an article called 'Gardasil: What lack of informed consent did for me', which was published on the Sanevax website <http://sanevax.org/gardasil-lack-informed-consent/>.

She says:

I had seen many Gardasil commercials on television and wanted to be 'one less girl' affected by cervical cancer. My doctor said I needed the HPV vaccine and I trusted the information I was given. I believed the vaccine was important for my health. I chose to get vaccinated. I had never taken the time to research Gardasil, or any other vaccines. I believed vaccines were simply a part of the 'healthcare' system; a system I trusted. I did not know vaccinating while your immune system was compromised could exacerbate the risks of adverse vaccine reaction.

Nicole was given her first Gardasil injection at a regular gynae-cological check-up. Her previous health conditions included some spinal issues and associated pain.

Within the first few days and for the week after the Gardasil shot, I was bedridden, sick with what we thought was a bad flu. It was also possible I was having a reaction from the muscle relaxer withdrawal or the side effects of my newly prescribed birth control pills. I stopped taking the birth control pills after eight days and my symptoms worsened.

My mother and fiancé remember the physical changes when I wasn't feeling well, but those few days after Gardasil have blurred together for me. I was so sick. During the days, weeks and months to come, I experienced the worst nausea, weakness, vomiting, and most severe pain in every crevice of my stomach and body that I have ever felt in my life. Even the other stomach sensitivities and spinal issues I had experienced previously absolutely paled in comparison to what happened to me after getting Gardasil.

We went to every doctor appointment and tested everything we possibly could. The tests kept coming back 'normal'. (Ironically, they never tested for metal poisoning, which I expressed symptoms of. If any doctor would have known those symptoms, I had nearly all of them, perhaps I wouldn't have suffered for so long.) None of the doctors said there could be any connection with Gardasil. In fact, most told us just the opposite; that my symptoms were definitely not caused by Gardasil … Within a month of my only Gardasil vaccination I was a completely changed, debilitated human being (Alexandra, 2014).

The introduction of Gardasil was heralded as the first ever anti-cancer vaccine and preceded by an intense marketing campaign built on fear (see Chapter 7). As previously discussed, it is still unknown if Gardasil will prevent a single case of cervical cancer. And yet, as these case studies and many others available on the Sanevax website show, Gardasil can have serious adverse effects including death.

The question we need to ask is if the young women and men who receive this vaccine have fully consented prior to the injection(s). Such consent would need to spell out a) the lack of evidence of prevention of cervical cancer to date and b) documented adverse effects including deaths. It would ensure that all recipients of Gardasil understand why the vaccine is being given and are fully informed of the potential risks of the procedure.

Informed consent prior to any medical intervention is a basic human right. This right has not been extended to the young women and men who have died nor to those who have been damaged by this experimental vaccine. We must make sure that the voices of victims are heard and that young women and men are told of the risks of HPV vaccines before they receive the injection(s).

Informed consent means that parents of girls and boys must be given the facts on the risks and supposed benefits of HPV vaccines. This also includes being told that Australian women are not at great risk of dying from cervical cancer. (As mentioned earlier, according to the Cancer Council Australia in 2014, 223 Australian women died as a result of cervical cancer (Cancer Council Australia, 2016a). This compares to 2,892 deaths from breast cancer in Australia (30 males and 2,862 females) in 2013 (Cancer Australia, 2017a) and 4,162 deaths from bowel cancer in 2013 (Cancer Australia, 2017b). Having the ability to make an informed decision about a medical intervention such as Gardasil means being aware that there are other ways of remaining free from cervical cancer such as having a healthy lifestyle (see p. 13) and undergoing regular Pap smears which enable early detection and treatment.

Gardasil was tested on fewer than 1,200 girls under the age of 16 (National Vaccine Information Center, NVIC, 2007). And yet in Australia, all girls as young as 12 are encouraged to be vaccinated through school-based programs. This information should form part of any informed consent procedure as should the information that the manufacturer Merck was able to use a placebo containing aluminium as a control, rather than a non-reactive saline solution placebo in the trials. Use of a reactive placebo such as aluminium can artificially increase the appearance of safety of an experimental drug or vaccine in a clinical trial. Being fully informed would also mean that recipients are aware that Gardasil and Gardasil 9 contain high levels of aluminium. Studies have shown that aluminium can result in nerve cell death and that vaccine aluminium adjuvants enable aluminium to enter the brain (NVIC, 2006).

For Nicole and many other young people suffering severe adverse reactions after HPV vaccinations, this information was not provided:

> I was not told that regular pap smears were an effective way to detect abnormal cells which could be treated before they developed into cervical cancer. I was not told the vast majority of HPV infections would clear up on their own with no health consequences. I was not given adequate information about the adverse reactions that could occur after Gardasil. I wish I had known then what I know now (Alexandra, 2014).

In spite of the lack of informed consent and the growing number of documented serious adverse vaccine reactions, Gardasil and Gardasil 9 (as well as Cervarix) continue to be rolled out. In fact it looks as if the consumer group might even be increased. It is extremely worrying to read that a new clinical trial is to look at the effects of the HPV vaccine Gardasil in *infants*. The clinical trial is called *4-valent HPV Vaccine to Treat Recurrent Respiratory Papillomatosis in Children* (U.S. National Institutes of Health, 2013). As the National Organization for Rare Diseases (NORD) notes: "Recurrent respiratory papillomatosis (RRP) is a rare disorder characterised by the development of small, wart-like growths (papillomas) in the respiratory tract" (NORD, 2016).

USA based researcher, writer and activist Marcella Piper-Terry has long-feared Gardasil might be added to the infant vaccine schedule. To think that babies may be next in line for this vaccine is extremely troublesome. Piper-Terry explains that the idea is to protect babies from respiratory infections. Gardasil contains two strains 6 and 11 said to be associated with recurrent respiratory infections (Piper-Terry, 2016).

We really need to ask why extending the target groups for HPV vaccines to even younger children is under consideration when we already know that HPV vaccines are associated with the highest number of reported adverse effects of any vaccine (Fisher, 2009b). Young children's lives that start out full of promise would be at risk after injections with these genetically engineered vaccines that contain large amounts of aluminium and other potentially harmful substances.

Chapter 7: The Marketing of Gardasil

> The mythology surrounding viruses is deeply misleading. They are frequently targeted and described as intelligent enemies that deserve to have a multi-billion dollar 'war on terror' waged against them to the great benefit of the pharmaceutical industry.
>
> — Janine Roberts, *Fear of the Invisible: How scared should we be of Viruses and Vaccines, HIV and Aids* (Roberts, 2008, p. 258)

In June 2006, the Therapeutic Goods Administration (TGA) approved the use of Gardasil in Australia for females aged nine to 26 and males aged nine to 15. The national HPV vaccination program began in 2007 and was provided free in schools for females aged 12–13 years (*Sydney Morning Herald*, 2006). This free program was extended to males aged 12–13 years in 2013.

The HPV vaccine was approved for use in Australia on the basis that it would prevent cervical cancer despite the fact that Australia has one of the lowest rates of cervical cancer in the world. Gardasil is today authorised for use in 130 countries and 205 million doses have been administered. Gardasil still dominates the global market for HPV vaccines bringing in profits of more than US $1 billion a year (Uniquest, 2016).[17]

---

17 Uniquest is the main commercialisation company of the University of Queensland (Uniquest, 2014).

The roll-out of Gardasil was preceded by years of promotion by the manufacturer Merck (USA) and CSL Ltd, the New Zealand and Australian distributor culminating in a relentless propaganda campaign waged by both Australian and international mass media. It started in the late 1990s with stories such as 'Dangerous Liaisons', published in the *Los Angeles Times Magazine*.

> Patty and Victor were infected with a strain of HPV — the virus that lurks behind one of the country's fastest-spreading, sexually transmitted diseases and is rapidly becoming a prime suspect in the search for the causes of cervical cancer … What's more, some people are spreading the virus unknowingly: It is transmitted by contact with warts, and warts go unnoticed. Some physicians suspect that HPV may even occasionally be spread indirectly — perhaps on a tanning bed, toilet or washcloth (Scott, 1990).

Prior to the 2006 release of Gardasil in the USA, the media message was intense and scarcely a day passed without a cervical cancer story accompanied by the promotion of an auspicious, imminent vaccine. This message reached an uninformed public, most of whom had never heard of this virus but were now anxiously waiting for a vaccine to become available as quickly as possible.

In *Vaccine Nation: America's Changing Relationship with Immunization* (2014), Elena Conis states that studies done during the early 2000s found that most US women had never heard of HPV and only half of those who knew about it were aware of the potential link to cervical cancer (p. 237). Conis describes one of the many advertisements that ran before and during popular American TV shows starring young, strong, healthy, athletic and good-looking girls riding horses, playing soccer, dancing and swimming, all united by the one cause: "to be one less victim of cervical cancer" (Conis, 2014, p. 236). Indeed 'One Less' became the slogan for Gardasil known throughout the world (Gardasil Commercial 2006).

In *The Guardian*, Sarah Boseley reported that public health experts such as Britain's Angela Raffle referred to the tactics used by the drug companies as "a battering ram at the Department of Health and carpet bombing on the peripheries" (Boseley, 2007). Dr Raffle was one of many experts that the British pharmaceutical companies attempted to recruit by offering to help her plan the introduction of the vaccine. She received countless letters from sales representatives eager to assist her to introduce the vaccine. But one of Raffle's chief concerns was that the emphasis on mass vaccination would damage the well-established successful screening programs. Sadly her fears were not misplaced for in Australia from December 2017, an HPV test will replace the Pap smear test as the first line of defence in the prevention of cervical cancer, followed, quite possibly, by an increased rate of vaccination with HPV vaccines. (See Chapter 3 for more details on this policy change.)

Those of us who have followed this story closely are not likely to forget the Australian media's love affair with our own Professor Ian Frazer who along with Dr Jian Zhou and others developed Gardasil. The *Sydney Morning Herald* science journalist Leigh Dayton filed one of the many confident interviews given by the Scottish-born Australian scientist Ian Frazer (Dayton, 1997, p. 5):

Cervical Cancer Vaccine Getting Closer

Researchers worldwide are closing in on vaccines against the virus that causes cervical cancer, a leading expert claims.

Dr Ian Frazer, an immunologist with the University of Queensland and Princess Alexandra Hospital in Brisbane, said the vaccines, now being tested on people, would target the human papillomavirus HPV, especially HPV16. 'It is now widely acknowledged as the cause of cervical cancer,' Dr Frazer said: 'So if we knock off HPV, we'll knock off cervical cancer.'

Long-term women's health researcher Renate Klein explains that one of the reasons for the successful marketing of the vaccine in Australia, was due to 'a good dose of patriotism' (Klein, 2008). The Australian public was given to believe that Queensland scientist, Professor Ian Frazer, along with his colleague Dr Jian Zhou were the sole inventors of the HPV vaccine. Subsequently Ian Frazer became a national hero and even the Australian of the Year in 2006.

There are many who believe that too much credit has been given to Ian Frazer. Robert Rose, associate professor of medicine at the University of Rochester in New York stated:

To say that the vaccine was developed in Ian's laboratory is a stretch in the papillomavirus research community. We certainly don't want to take away from the sense of pride that Australia has in Ian's work, but it's not really correct in our view to see the vaccine as something he invented (in Beran, 2006).

The University of Rochester is one of four research institutions claiming responsibility for the original work leading to a cervical cancer vaccine along with the US National Cancer Institute

(NCI), Georgetown University in Washington DC, and the University of Queensland. According to Robert Rose, "Frazer allowed the perception to grow that he was the sole inventor of the vaccine and that's not accurate." None of this was of great concern to Ian Frazer: "We're going to get a vaccine. The vaccine will be of benefit to women. Who invented it probably doesn't matter very much" (in Beran, 2006).

But was it Ian Frazer and his partner Jian Zhou who were the first to invent and lodge the patent, or was it one of the other institutions from the USA? In her biography of Ian Frazer, Madonna King (2013) explores this question and the subsequent wrangle and ensuing court hearings. Much depended on the result with US manufacturer Merck growing increasingly worried. Merck was due to announce its new vaccine Gardasil. The University of Queensland where Frazer had worked since 1985 was aware that it might lose out on significant profits. The decision made by the United States Patent and Trademark Office was finally reached in 2005 stating that Ian Frazer and Jian Zhou were not the first to make HPV virus-like particles (VLPs). This decision was based on the belief that they had not used the wild HPV16 L1 Protein in the production of the VLP and therefore would not be awarded the patent. The prize instead went to Georgetown University. King writes: "Ian Frazer had shown little emotion when told of the verdict" (King 2013, p. 133). The vaccine was on its way and he had more research to do. But in 2006, an appeal of the 2005 patent decision was lodged. This was at the same time as the media began to focus on Ian Frazer as the 'Australian of the Year' and Merck was releasing Gardasil in the US. And this time the US Court of Appeals announced that the patent belonged to the University of Queensland (King, 2013). In making this decision, one of the factors that the court took into consideration was that Ian Frazer and Jian Zhou had presented their work at an HPV conference in 1991 and the knowledge on how to produce the VLP was therefore imparted to others (King 2013, p. 138).

Madonna King does not neglect to mention the huge financial gains that were to be made from the patent win.

> By the end of 2012, the vaccine globally had provided revenue to CSL of six hundred million dollars. A slice of that is then divided into thirds between The University of Queensland's commercial arm, UniQuest, and The University of Queensland's Diamantina Institute, and the final third is shared equally between Ian and the estate of Jian Zhou (p. 139).

But in spite of the financial success and the fanfare that accompanied the launch of Gardasil, as we now know there is no proof that HPV vaccines will prevent cervical cancer.

The prominent role played by the media in the marketing of Gardasil did not pass unnoticed with a pro-business media watchdog group finding in 2008 that the hype wasn't the result of over-the-top marketing by Merck, but was instead the result of heavy promotion by the American news media.

In *Blaming the Media for Gardasil Hype*, Tara Parker Hope (2008) cites many examples:

- NBC's Brian Williams called Gardasil a "triumph in science and medicine" referring to it as "the first vaccine to prevent cancer" and urging parents to get their children vaccinated.

- NBC's 'Today' show co-host Meredith Vieira declared that it "could save your teenager's life someday." She also told viewers Gardasil was one of the three vaccines kids "need."
- For 'The Early Show' on CBS, Dr Emily Senay stated that the "top medical breakthrough [of 2006] has to be the cancer vaccine for cervical cancer, Gardasil."

Behind the Australian Gardasil campaign was the PR giant Edelman that worked with the Australian and New Zealand distributor CSL Biotherapies in promoting the vaccine to health professionals and the public. There were 974 pieces of media devoted to the campaign with over 40 hours of coverage available to the Australian audience of almost 24 million. The campaign engaged 21 women between the ages of 14–26 who were to be given the vaccination nationally. Gardasil was launched to the public on 28 August 2006 and Ian Frazer himself vaccinated the first woman at the Sydney launch. The media campaign resulted in over 60% of mothers recommending their daughters avail themselves of the vaccination. More than 50% of women had now become aware of the vaccine with general practitioners reporting they had around eight patients requesting information about the drug (Public Relations Institute of Australia, PRIA, 2007).

Documenting how Gardasil was sold to the public would not be complete without the inclusion of the role played by commercial interests such as CSL Ltd, the Australian and New Zealand distributor of Gardasil, and that of Australian politics. In 'Healthcare's sticking point', Gina McColl describes how the listing of anti-cancer vaccines such as Gardasil highlights how commercial pressure and politics threaten the independence of our healthcare system. In November 2006, CSL's first application for listing Gardasil on the national immunisation register was declined by the Pharmaceutical Benefits Advisory Committee (PBAC).[18]

Tony Abbott, who was Minister for Health at the time, defended this decision, but due to an intense public outcry, Prime Minister John Howard stepped in, promising the electorate that the vaccine would be approved (McColl, 2007).

Writing for *The Australian*, Matthew Stevens sums up the political manoeuvre:

> It took just 24 hours for the then Australian Prime Minister, John Howard, to put an end to the nonsense, delivering sparkling prime ministerial endorsement to Gardasil along with a clear direction to Minister Abbott that the immunisation program should proceed. And pronto (Stevens, 2006).

Those critical of the HPV vaccination program were furious. Activist Elizabeth Hart described the significance of John Howard's interference in the PBAC's initial application:

> Getting a vaccine on the national schedule must be the 'golden goose' for vaccine manufacturers as this assures a mass market for their vaccine product. It also helps create a 'domino' effect as other countries follow suit and adopt the vaccine, creating a mass global market (Hart, 2013).

---

18 The PBAC is an independent expert body appointed by the Australian Government. Its primary role is to recommend new medicines for listing on the Pharmaceutical Benefits Scheme (PBS, 2016).

And so it came to pass that on International Women's Day, March 8th 2007, the then federal Minister for Health Tony Abbott announced to the Australian people that the cervical cancer vaccination program was set to begin.

Opposition to Gardasil continues to grow with U.S. blogger Dr Kelly Brogan articulating the feelings of so many of us who have watched with disappointment the introduction of HPV vaccines to uninformed young girls:

> … the Pharmaceutical industry has co-opted our maternal inner compass. They, in partnership with media, have grabbed onto our natural tendency to worry about the welfare of our children, and they have tempted us with a shiny apple. Visiting again and again until we relent … Every day, in my office, I have women expressing poignant remorse, shame, and rage because they trusted their Pharma-pushing doctor instead of trusting themselves, trusting in the inherent potential of the body to be well, to heal, to surmount seeming obstacles. No cohort of women are more lionized than those who have lost their daughters to a vaccine promoted to save them from a disease they were never going to get (Brogan, 2015).

The mainstream media has failed in its duty to inform the public that there are serious problems with the 'HPV-causes-cervical-cancer' hypothesis. Australia has one of the lowest rates of cervical cancer in the world. The incidence rate of cervical cancer in Australia is 6.8 per 100,000 women and the incidence rate of mortality is 1.7 per 100,000 women (Cancer Australia, 2017d). Around 80% of the women in Australia and other developed countries are exposed or have been exposed to HPV, and yet fewer than 1% of all women in these countries will be diagnosed with cervical cancer. If the journalists had done their research they would have also learnt that 90% of HPV infections resolve themselves naturally within a year according to Diane Harper, one of the developers of Gardasil.

Diane Harper has many damning things to say about the vaccine she helped to create. Amongst them is this shocking statement:

> The rate of serious adverse events (from Gardasil) is on par with the death rate of cervical cancer. Gardasil has been associated with at least as many serious adverse events as there are deaths from cervical cancer developing each year (Harper in Renter, 2013).

It is indeed questionable if young girls need a vaccine against HPV because the majority of these infections clear up by themselves. Cervical cancer is still a serious disease but its incidence has markedly decreased over the last few decades especially in Western countries because of improvements in living standards and the success of Pap smear programs. In developing nations where women are still at a high risk of cervical cancer it is time to address the issues of poverty and inequality making them more susceptible to ill health (see also pp. 99–102) for the scandalous Gardasil trials that were conducted on poor Indian tribal girls).

Chapter 8: Dissent

> The strongest bulwark of authority is uniformity; the least divergence from it is the greatest crime.
>
> — Emma Goldman
> (in Shulman, 1996)

It is crucial to speak out about adverse events associated with HPV vaccines. Since the introduction of Gardasil in 2006 in the USA, there have been over 50,000 documented adverse effects and 315 deaths according to the Vaccine Adverse Event Reporting System or VAERS (SaneVax, Inc., 2017). My own attempt to make sense of this mass vaccination program began in 2005, before the introduction of Gardasil to Australian girls. I wrote an article called 'The Politics of Pap Smears', which was published by the online magazine *New Matilda* (Lobato, 2005). In this piece I suggested that we did not need a vaccine to treat cervical cancer because there was no evidence of a direct causal relationship between HPV and cervical cancer. I pointed out that while HPV infection is extremely common, very few women develop cervical cancer. In fact the incidence of cervical cancer in all women is about 1% (Duesberg and Schwartz, 1992).

I have continued my opposition to HPV vaccination and have written many passionate letters to the editors of various newspapers. On one occasion I wrote a letter to the mainstream papers penned in response to the announcement that all was set for the cervical cancer vaccination campaign to begin. However this letter was not published by any of the popular press outlets (Lobato, 2007). I argued that Australia should not be vaccinating young girls with a vaccine to protect them from the human papilloma virus when there has been no conclusive proof that the HPV virus causes all cervical cancers.

I wished to point out that as with all cancers, the dynamics of cervical cancer development does not match the behaviour of viruses. Papilloma viruses cause papillomas or warts on young sexually active adults. These small (over)growths of slightly abnormal cells can appear and disappear almost overnight and are not malignant. On the other hand, cervical cancers develop from benign hyperplasias or excessive growths of nearly normal cervical tissue. Most of these disappear and only some cells on the cervix undergo abnormal changes (dysplasia) which can then go on to become cancerous.

The major feature of cancer progression is that it is irregular and gradual — quite unlike the rapid and consistent development of warts. Perhaps a more likely explanation for the development of these cancers can be found when we examine the known risks or co-factors for the disease which should not be overlooked. Wang *et al*. point to the fact that HPV is now accepted as the necessary but not sufficient cause for cervical neoplasia or cancer. They found that HPV co-factors for cervical cancer include smoking, multiparity (having given birth to more than one child) and oral contraceptive use (Wang *et al*., 2009). This point is supported by the work of Kirsten Jensen *et al*. who studied the effect of a woman's reproductive history on the risk of developing pre-cancerous lesions and concluded that childbirth increased the risk, and particularly so in women with persistent high-risk HPV infection (Jensen *et al.*, 2013). Very little attention is paid to these co-factors that may make some women more vulnerable to cancer. Some of these co-factors exist because of adverse social, environmental and economic factors that frequently accompany women's lives. Equal access to a nourishing diet that is protective against cancer is not available to all women. Neither is information about the disease and how to avoid it generally accessible.

Over the months and years that followed I continued to speak out about the problems with, and dangers of, HPV vaccination and was joined by many like-minded people. Feminist health researchers, parents of young girls harmed by the vaccines, and others concerned about the vaccines were expressing their concerns by establishing newsletters and blogs. One of these blogs was *Gardasil: Women Hurt By Medicine*, edited by a student of politics and the media, Gertrude Green, together with biologist and social scientist Dr Renate Klein. Both were very concerned about these vaccines calling them "a gigantic experiment on women's bodies" (Green and Klein, 2008). They devoted their blog to women's own stories about cervical cancer vaccines and to gathering background information.[19] Shortly after the government funded administration of the Gardasil vaccine to

---

19 <https://womenhurtbymedicine.wordpress.com> The blog remains accessible and has a lot of background information on the Gardasil saga in addition to stories that affected young women posted, especially from Australia. It stopped being updated when SaneVax started their website in 2010 in order to avoid duplication.

Australian girls began in April 2007, Renate Klein, and author and commentator Melinda Tankard Reist, warned that "the much trumpeted inject-every-girl-free-with-Gardasil campaign has run into a bit of a snag." Their 2007 article published on the social and public debate website *On Line Opinion* broadcast the news that four Melbourne schoolgirls were rushed to hospital after receiving the vaccine. Sixteen other girls were reported sick and one student was left paralysed for six hours. This was dismissed by CSL, the Australian and New Zealand distributor of Gardasil as due to 'stress' and 'anxiety'. Klein and Tankard Reist revealed that deaths after having received the HPV vaccine had occurred in the USA and asserted that Australian girls who receive the vaccine "are taking part in what is really a major experiment" (Klein and Tankard Reist, 2007).

Renate Klein has continued her strong opposition to this large-scale experiment carried out on the bodies of young girls and now boys. In a later article, again published by *On Line Opinion*, she warned that Gardasil vaccinations could be associated with anaphylaxis, seizures, unremitting tiredness, chest pain, body rashes, problems with mobility, and menstrual pain and irregularities. Klein also warned that many young girls were developing serious neurological diseases such as Guillain-Barré Syndrome, and Acute Demyelinating Encephalomyelitis. There were also unexplained reports of miscarriages post vaccination and of foetal abnormalities appearing in the offspring of women who were mistakenly given the vaccine when they were pregnant.

Furious, Klein called for the then Minister for Health, Nicola Roxon, to suspend the Gardasil vaccination program before it claimed more victims and demanded a thorough investigation into the health of vaccine recipients (Klein, 2008). Roxon and other politicians were directly approached by other activists, but they never responded. Meanwhile, the mainstream media has been woefully silent about the harm from this vaccine.

Over the past nine years, the 'fourth estate' has been repeatedly approached and fed the harrowing stories of injury and death in association with Gardasil vaccinations, but with some rare exceptions, they have refused to publish them.

Stephen Tunley is a committed activist warning people both in Australia and globally about the life-changing side effects of HPV vaccines. The Sydney businessman is also a Director of SaneVax Inc. an international organisation of dedicated individuals whose primary goal is to provide information to the general public in order for people to make informed decisions regarding their health and wellbeing. In 2009, Tunley's healthy daughter had become seriously ill and suffered seizures, tremors and tachycardia (an abnormally fast resting heart beat) after her second Gardasil injection. Like so many other unfortunate young women post Gardasil, the 19-year-old has continued to be in poor health. In August 2011, prompted by a Channel Nine *60 Minutes* program called *Getting the Point*,[20] a program about vaccination, Tunley wrote to the producers suggesting that they might like

20 *Getting the Point* by reporter Ellen Fanning on *60 Minutes* (Fanning, 2011). Vaccine researcher Judy Wilyman had this to say about the program: This program did not provide a balanced presentation of the vaccination issue. It also did not allow for discussion or debate of the issues presented. It relied on the program directors selecting the script for the program and selecting the comments they wanted from the interviewees (Wilyman, 2011).

to run a second program giving "the other story where young women, their parents and GPs talk about the dirty side of 'fear marketed' vaccines" (Tunley, 2011). Channel Nine did not take up his suggestion. Stephen has also written to the ABC, SBS, the 7.30 program (ABC-TV) and many other media outlets, but no program has ever eventuated. He has alerted politicians, medical associations and regulators asking for them to review their health policies in regard to the HPV vaccines. He is still waiting.

Stephen Tunley explains this lack of responsiveness:

> Fact is that with a regulator (TGA) wholly funded by those it administers, with a Government in the thrall of big corporations, with media under the thrall of the political interests of its owners, with Universities and teaching hospitals reliant on funding from Pharma the issues do not get an airtime (Tunley, 2016).

Fortunately, since 2010, we now have access to the SaneVax website where we can continue to read heartfelt stories of girls who have suffered adverse health events in the wake of Gardasil. In doing the job that the mainstream media should be doing, the dedicated SaneVax organisers detail the trauma of those who never recover their former health because they or their parents thought they were doing the right thing in agreeing to the HPV vaccinations (SaneVax, Inc. 2017a).

SaneVax began publishing after the President, Norma Erickson, and the Secretary, Freda Birrell were stunned by the stories they were hearing of girls becoming ill after Gardasil. They wanted to do all they could to help the survivors. They created their website with the assistance of a group of like-minded individuals, some of whom had HPV vaccine-injured children themselves.

Other committed dissenters include Australian Judy Wilyman who began researching vaccination after her first child was vaccinated in 1993 (Wilyman, 2016). Wilyman is the publisher of the 'Vaccination Decision' newsletter found on her website Vaccination Decisions (Wilyman, 2016) (<http://vaccinationdecisions.net>). In 2015, she completed her PhD thesis 'A critical analysis of the Australian Government's rationale for its vaccination policy' in which she devotes a detailed chapter to HPV and cervical cancer (Wilyman, 2015). Wilyman is tireless in her efforts to inform a long list of politicians and media outlets about her research into vaccination, but is usually met with stony silence.

After many years of research into cervical cancer and the continuous search for a cause of this disease, I have come to the conclusion that resistance to Gardasil needs to include an alternative explanation of the development of cancer in the human body. A holistic understanding of the dreaded Big 'C' is required, one that questions whether cancer can be caused by viruses, thus eliminating the rationale to use vaccines such as Gardasil. Perhaps such an enlightened clarification would include an appreciation of cancer as a 'biological phenomenon' (Adams, 2015) as suggested by Professor Paul Davies.[21] Davies is a cosmologist and physicist who now works at the Centre for Convergence of Physical Science and Cancer Biology at Arizona

---

21 'Cancer can teach us about our own evolution' an opinion article by Paul Davies (Davies, 2012).

State University. Around nine years ago, the then deputy director of the United States National Cancer Institute called on his skills as a physicist to be used for cancer research. Speaking with radio broadcaster Phillip Adams on *Late Night Live* in 2015, Paul Davies explained that as we age we develop many small tumours but that the body mostly manages to hold these in check. "Cancer is part of the way that multicellular life works," Davies said, adding that "everyone" has cancer, but in most cases it never becomes clinically relevant: the body just deals with it.

Davies claims that most cancer biologists are thinking about the problem the wrong way round and that the questions that researchers should be asking are: What is cancer for? Where does cancer fit into this story of life?

Davies calls for an alternative approach to cancer because, as he explains it, there are trillions of dollars invested in cancer research and yet the mortality rates have hardly changed. The U.S. National Cancer Institute spends about $US5 billion a year on cancer research (in Strom, 2015). But, sadly, all these miracle drugs have only prolonged life — often just weeks, perhaps months, rarely years. Professor Davies calls it the "lure of the cure" (Adams, 2015).

If he is correct and cancer is "part of the logic of life" where does that leave the HPV-equals-cervical-cancer theory including the need for HPV vaccines? And where will atonement for the damage to young girls and women come from?

Chapter 9: Resistance

> At 12 years old, my beautiful daughter
> Jemma was a happy, bright, fun-loving girl
> filled with energy. She was always on the go,
> never content to just sit around the house.
> Jemma was continuously asking to go to a
> friend's place for a sleep-over or arranging to
> be entertained by other activities. I decided
> to allow Jemma to have the HPV vaccine,
> Gardasil. This had a huge impact for me.
> My whole soul was riddled with guilt. I felt it
> was the worst decision I had ever made for
> my child and certainly my biggest regret ever.
> I can't tell you how many times the phrase
> IF ONLY, IF ONLY... echoed through my
> mind!!!! As the years have passed, I have
> been somewhat able to overcome this.
> Now, I concentrate my energy on the
> healing process for my daughter
>
> — (Jenny, 2016)

Over 205 million doses of Gardasil had been distributed globally to July 2016. In Australia, with about 9 million Gardasil doses distributed, and with over 3,905 reports of adverse events up to December 2016 (Therapeutic Goods Administration, 2017), there has been no move by health authorities to question or withdraw support for the HPV vaccines. Other nations have taken steps to address the harm done to young women and men, acting in response to urgent calls from activists and the general public for health policies to address the interests of the people, rather than those of Big Pharma.

While the HPV vaccines are currently approved for use in more than 130 countries, in Japan, Spain and France criminal lawsuits have been filed. In June 2013, the Japanese government withdrew its recommendation for the human papillomavirus (HPV) vaccines to be given to young girls aged 12–16 due to concerns from the public over adverse effects. This precautionary move followed reports of 1,968 cases of possible adverse effects including body pain, numbness and paralysis (see Klein and Lobato, 2013). A special task force examined 43 cases of widespread pain after HPV vaccinations reporting that a connection between the adverse events and HPV vaccines could not be ruled out. Japan hasn't gone as far as banning the vaccines but its government has withdrawn support for the program and insists that doctors be required to inform girls of its position. Interestingly, since the Japanese government withdrew its support in 2013, the HPV vaccination rate has fallen from 70% to 1% of girls (Zielinski, 2016).

In July 2016, 63 Japanese women and girls aged between 15 to 22 years sued the government and the drug makers GlaxoSmithKline PLC of Britain and Merck Sharp and Dohme Corp. a subsidiary of U.S. giant Merck and Co., for damages over health problems they suffered after they were vaccinated with the HPV vaccines Cervarix and Gardasil. The plaintiffs who had experienced a range of health problems starting after their HPV vaccines are seeking compensation of at least 15 million yen each. The women insist that the government provide expert medical help for their symptoms and that research for a cure happens (Otake, 2016). The lawsuit is unlikely to be decided quickly and will depend on the level of proof submitted by the plaintiffs. However, the women's lawyers have stated: "the causal relationship will be acknowledged because the victims have common symptoms"(Jiji, 2016). Meanwhile, the government hopes to use a new survey of hospital patients to ascertain how many patients who haven't been vaccinated with HPV vaccines also developed these symptoms in order to find out if a causal relationship exists. The survey is expected to have a bearing on the case and will also be used in deciding whether the government changes its recommendation for HPV vaccination of its citizens (Jiji, 2016).

While the Australian government has been woefully silent on Gardasil, it has been up to sick women themselves to attempt to get justice. In 2013, Naomi Snell, a 28-year-old Melbourne woman, began a class action civil lawsuit against drug maker Merck after suffering autoimmune and neurological complications following her Gardasil shots. Her disabling symptoms included convulsions, severe back and neck pain, and an inability to walk. This caused her doctors to suspect she had multiple sclerosis, a diagnosis that was later retracted in favour of a neurological reaction to the vaccine. Seven other women, who had also been very ill following their HPV vaccinations, joined Naomi in her battle to seek justice (Gucciardi, 2011). However, the claim against Merck did not proceed as the litigant Naomi was suffering considerable stress brought on by the impending case. According to an article in the *Waverley Leader*, Naomi Snell became very ill and decided to put her health first (Schmidt, 2011).

Meanwhile, concern over HPV vaccines is increasing all over the world. In June 2014, Spanish Attorney Don Manuel Sáez Ochoa filed a complaint against Merck-Sanofi Pasteur Laboratories, Spanish National Health authorities, and the regional health authorities of the La Rioja province for its failure to use an inert placebo[22] when trialling the vaccines "thereby manipulating data and of marketing Gardasil under false pretences" (Erickson, 2014a). A moratorium that was called for until safety issues were determined went unheeded.

In France, calls for a parliamentary inquiry into HPV vaccines resulted in a petition signed by more than 700 doctors and 300 midwives who argued that the vaccines' effectiveness remains to be proven (La Vigne, 2015). Criminal complaints have been filed in France on behalf of 10 young women who have been suffering autoimmune disorders after they had their Gardasil shots (Erickson 2013).

In Ireland, the parents of girls from the group REGRET (Reactions and Effects of Gardasil Resulting in Extreme Trauma) met with members of the health department who listened to the

---

22 The placebo used was aluminium hydroxide, a chemical substance which, when added to a vaccine, provokes a reaction. A placebo should be a totally inert substance such as normal saline that doesn't provoke an immune response. The fact that there are not more reactions in the group which received the vaccine than in those who received the 'placebo', does not make the vaccine safe (see also p. 70).

stories of the girls' conditions but concluded that the vaccine wasn't at fault (TV3, 2015). Three hundred women are diagnosed with cervical cancer each year in Ireland and 100 women die from it. Gardasil vaccinations began in Ireland in 2010. By now REGRET has information from 150 girls who have become severely unwell after receiving HPV vaccines. Laura is one of the Irish 'Gardasil Girls'. She was a normal active teenager and an "asset in the classroom," said her mother. After her first Gardasil shot, Laura became unwell and required her mother to pick her up from school. When she complained of dizziness, headache and nausea, she was told this was normal. Her condition worsened after her second vaccination to such an extent that she soon was unable to attend school. According to her doctors, she was suffering chronic fatigue syndrome but whatever the authorities chose to call their debilitating conditions, the girls and their families are united in their conviction that they became ill after their HPV vaccinations (TV3 Ireland, 2016). The parents are very angry that they were not told about the extent of the possible adverse effects when they signed the vaccination consent form. With the heavy toll on young women and boys' health and indeed the public purse that funds these vaccination programs in countries like Australia, there are more calls for a moratorium on the vaccinations until further studies are conducted.

At a meeting held in order to debate Gardasil and Cervarix, Michèle Rivasi, a French member of the European Parliament, opened with the following comment:

> These vaccines are unnecessary, dangerous to many, and certainly a huge drain on precious public health funds. To halt HPV vaccination

programs, pending intense investigation and proof of stated purpose could very well be the salvation of our young people (in Erickson, 2014a).

Urgent calls for an inquiry from campaigners in Britain, Denmark and Sweden were finally heeded and in July 2015, the European Medicines Agency (EMA) announced a review into two of the adverse conditions: complex regional pain syndrome CRPS[23] and postural orthostatic tachycardia syndrome POTS.[24]

However, despite hearing details of damaged girls from countries including Spain, Italy, France, Colombia and Mexico submitted by the Asociacion de Afectadas por la Vacuna del Papiloma (AAVP), the Association of women affected by HPV vaccines, the committee could see no reason to change the way the vaccines were administered, or the need to amend the current product information. Indeed, the EMA claimed that the benefits of HPV vaccines continue to outweigh their risks (in Capilla, 2015).

Following the EMA's handling of this important issue, criticism came from other quarters including the Nordic

---

23 CRPS is a chronic pain condition occurring after damage to the peripheral and central nervous systems. Areas of the body most affected are arms, legs, hands, or feet (NIH, National Institute of Neurological Disorders and Stroke, 2017).

24 POTS is a disturbance of the autonomic nervous system manifesting in symptoms such as fatigue, sweating, tremor, anxiety, palpitation, exercise intolerance, light-headedness, and near collapse on upright posture (Agarwal *et al.*, 2007).

Cochrane Centre.[25] The Centre, a reputable independent research and information organisation, was far from satisfied that the safety of the HPV vaccines had been adequately dealt with.

Its complaint to the European Medicines Agency (EMA) cast serious doubt upon the methods of the EMA and its handling of this issue. The organisation accused the EMA of being more concerned with its own reputation and acting to insulate the vaccines from criticism at all costs because of its belief that they could save lives by preventing the development of cervical cancer. According to Peter C. Gøtzsche, the Director of the Nordic Cochrane Centre and Rigshospitalet Professor, at the University of Copenhagen and his colleagues, the report undertaken by the EMA failed to take seriously important data that implicated the HPV vaccine in the development of severe side effects. Amongst them were findings by the Uppsala Monitoring Centre[26] that the HPV vaccines resulted in a considerably higher risk of severe adverse effects than any other vaccine. They question whether the EMA has respected the rights of the community to know that there are concerns related to the safety of the HPV vaccines.

We find it unacceptable that the EMA in its official report did not make it clear that it allowed the drug companies to be their own judges when evaluating whether the vaccine is safe, particularly since

---

25 The Nordic Cochrane Centre is part of Cochrane, an international network of individuals and institutions which researches and reviews the effects of health care (Cochrane Nordic, 2017).

26 The Uppsala Monitoring Centre (UMC), located in Uppsala, Sweden, is an independent, not-for-profit foundation for international scientific research. It is closely associated with the World Health Organisation and is about achieving the safer use of medicines (Uppsala Monitoring Centre, 2017).

there is a huge amount of money at stake: The global expenditure so far on HPV vaccines can be roughly estimated at €25 billion. The EMA asked the companies to search for side effects of the vaccine in their own databases and did not check the companies' work for accuracy (Gøtzsche, p. 5).

Peter C Gøtzsche concludes:

> Some people will prefer to avoid the vaccine, even if the risk of serious harm is very small, and some will prefer screening instead. It is not within the powers of regulatory authorities to deny citizens' right to make informed choices about their own health by withholding important information. The citizens need honest information about the vaccine and the uncertainties related to it; not a paternalistic statement that all is fine based on a flawed EMA report (Gøtzsche, p. 17).

At such frustrating times we need to return to the basic truth at the heart of these disturbing developments. For that I turn to Barbara Loe Fisher, president of the National Vaccine Information Center (NVIC) based in the USA, who stated:

> So here's the bottom line: The Gardasil vaccine is supposed to prevent a sexually transmitted infection that is naturally cleared from the body within two years by the vast majority of people. Getting regular Pap smears can help prevent almost all cases of cervical cancer and death (Fisher, 2010).

Fisher reminds us that pharmaceutical companies have been rolling out vaccines for a common virus that usually does not cause problems in order to prevent a disease that can be diagnosed simply by Pap smears — with treatment given in the case of moderate dysplasia CIN 2 and severe dysplasia CIN 3 or carcinoma in situ (see pp. 18–19).

And yet, these vaccination programs continue, with Gardasil provided free in Australian schools to all males and females aged 12–13 years under the National HPV Vaccination Program. The take-up rate for these free vaccinations is generally very high. Recently a friend told me that in her grandson's year 7 class he was the only one out of 25 students who did not present for the Gardasil shots. His parents had not given consent to the vaccination of their son. They had done their research.

Sadly, the parents of thousands of girls who were vaccinated as part of an unethical trial in India were not informed about the risks of these vaccines. The trial was called a 'demonstration project' and run by the Indian unit of the Program for Appropriate Technology in Health (PATH)[27] (Sarojini N. B. *et al.*, p. 28, 2010). The 2009 project was a joint venture between ICMR, the Indian Council of Medical Research, and the state governments of Andra Pradesh and Gujarat, with support from the Bill and Melinda Gates Foundation (Sarojini N. B. *et al.*, p. 28, 2010a).

The project, which was confirmed by the Ministry of Health and Family Welfare in 2010 as a "post-licensure operational research study," was, in reality, a "Phase IV, post marketing, clinical trial" (Sama, 2010a). It involved the vaccination of about 30,000

---

27 PATH (formerly called the Program for Appropriate Technology in Health) is an international, nonprofit global health organization based in Seattle. Founded in 1977 with a focus on family planning, PATH soon broadened its purpose to work on a wide array of emerging and persistent global health issues in the areas of health technologies such as immunisation (PATH, 2017).

girls, aged between 10–14 years. The vaccines used were Gardasil and Cervarix. Women's health groups were alarmed at the trials and very concerned that the HPV vaccines had not been tested for safety and efficacy in the Indian population where adolescent girls are often malnourished. They conducted their own investigation and found that the young girls selected for the trial — many of them poor tribal girls — came from communities lacking the necessary health infrastructure such as Pap smear facilities and gynaecologists. These young adolescent girls had put their faith in the government, naively trusting it to do the right thing — in this case providing them with an expensive vaccine free of cost, to prevent cervical cancer. However, there was no informed consent process; they were not told that they were part of a clinical trial and that they had the right to refuse participation. In the rare cases where consent forms were used, there was no information regarding compensation, or about possible alternative treatments or risk management (Sarojini N. B. *et al.*, p. 28, 2010a).

The girls were also not informed that one of the possible and significant side effects of the vaccine might be infertility. Notwithstanding the fact that at least four girls died in Andhra Pradesh in India and two in Gujarat, also in India, and that many girls went on to suffer severe side effects (including anaphylactic shock, seizures and paralysis, motor neurone disease, and disorders of the immune system), there has been no follow-up monitoring by PATH. The deaths were attributed to other causes such as malaria or suicide.

On World Health Day, April 7, 2010, representatives from the following women's groups, Jan Swasthya Abhiyaan (JSA),

All India Democratic Women's Association (AIDWA), Sama —
Resource Group for Women and Health, and Saheli Women's
Resource Centre, held a press conference to raise their concern
and opposition to the HPV vaccination trials. They demanded
that all trials with HPV vaccines be suspended and an inquiry
into the deaths "dubbed as suicides" held (Sama, 2010b). They
also insisted that every girl vaccinated be given an independent
medical examination to assess any side effects of the drugs.

In their memorandum to the Minister of Health the activists
wrote: "The very nature of this project seems to be unethical and
violates all norms of conducting trials on human subjects" (Sama,
2010b).

In April 2010, the ICMR told the governments of Andhra
Pradesh and Gujarat to immediately suspend the cervical
cancer control vaccination program for girls (Pandey, 2012).
In the same year, due largely to the insistence of the activists,
the Indian Government held an inquiry into the study and
found "that there were many gross violations in the project with
respect to procedures for taking informed consent, inadequate
health facilities for dealing with adverse events and medical
emergencies" (SaneVax, Inc. 2013). A further finding in April
2013 by a committee appointed by India's parliament accused
PATH of violating clinical-testing norms:

> Its [PATH's] sole aim has been to promote the commercial interests
> of HPV vaccine manufacturers who would have reaped windfall
> profits had PATH been successful in getting the HPV vaccine in the
> Universal Immunization Program of the country (Vn, 2013).

All of this is of course cold comfort to the parents of 13-year-old Sarita Kudumula who only learnt that their daughter had taken part in a medical trial after she collapsed and died a few days after her Gardasil injection. Girls from tribal communities such as Sarita are obliged to attend government schools located away from their communities which increases their vulnerability to exploitative drug trials. India with its large population and lax rules and regulations has become a popular country for pharmaceutical companies to test their drugs (Buncombe and Lakhani, 2011).

This chapter has been an attempt to record some of the worldwide resistance to the HPV vaccination programs. Yet while countries such as Japan are no longer promoting the vaccines, China is about to commence HPV vaccination for the first time. In July 2016, The China Food and Drug Administration (CFDA) approved Cervarix as the HPV vaccine of choice for Chinese children and young women. Because China has not offered HPV vaccinations before, those who wished to be vaccinated have travelled to Hong Kong where all three current HPV vaccines are available (Yiwen, 2016). However, the proposed Chinese HPV vaccination program has its critics with Dr Sin Hang Lee, a leading pathologist, worried about the effects that the vaccines will have on Chinese women. In August 2016, he sent an open letter to the President of China, Xi Junping, and the Premier of China, Li Keqiang, asking for a delay in the scheduled HPV vaccination of Chinese children and young women aged from nine to 25.

In his letter, Dr Lee, a Chinese American who has practiced laboratory medicine in North America for more than 50 years, asked the President and Premier of China to delay the program until the risks versus benefits of mass HPV vaccination of Chinese children and young women were adequately evaluated by independent medical and scientific experts. In Lee's words:

1. There is zero scientific evidence that HPV vaccines have been proven to prevent a single case of cervical cancer in any country.
2. To promote the vaccine, GSK [GlaxoSmithKline] created an unnecessary cervical cancer scare to create a market based on fear and not fact.
3. Due to genetic difference the HPV vaccines which were originally developed and tested in South America may not work across diverse Chinese ethnic populations.
4. Long established and low cost cervical screening, not vaccination, is a proven safe and effective means of controlling cervical cancer and as such should be the number one health program, saving billions of dollars and countless lives.
5. HPV vaccination offers no added value to existing cervical cancer screening programs.
6. Globally there are tens of thousands of serious adverse reactions, including deaths, following HPV vaccination.
7. Vaccine manufacturers have inappropriately used their proprietary highly immunogenicity-enhancing aluminum adjuvant as the placebo in all clinical trials and to do so in effect masks the risk of HPV vaccines (in Erickson, 2016b).

GlaxoSmithKline expects that the vaccine will be launched in China in 2017 (GSK, 2016). There are around 143 million females in this age group in China. Sales of the Cervarix vaccine could generate over $64 billion for the manufacturer if the Chinese government goes ahead with the vaccination program (Erickson, 2016b).

At the time of writing (2017) the outcome of Dr Lee's letter was unknown, nor do we know if the HPV vaccinations have started.

Chapter 10:
HPV or individual karyotypes to blame?

> You may choose to look the other way,
> but you can never say again that you
> did not know.
>
> — William Wilberforce, addressing the
> English parliament prior to the vote
> on the Abolition Bill, 1789
> (Macat, 2016)

According to Norma Erickson and Peter Duesberg (2015), even after more than 25 years of research into the hypothesis that HPV causes cervical cancer, there are still no direct answers to the following questions:

1. Why would only one in 10,000 HPV-infected women develop cervical cancer?
2. Why would cervical cancers only develop 20 to 50 years after infection? In other words, why would the virus not cause cancers when it is biochemically active and causing warts, namely before it is neutralized by natural anti-viral immunity?
3. Why are cervical carcinomas individually very distinct from each other in terms of malignancy, drug-resistance, cell histology, as originally described by Papanicolaou *et al.* in *Science* in 1952, although they are presumably caused by the same viral proteins?
4. Why are cervical carcinomas that are presumably generated by Human Papillomavirus proteins not immunogenic and thus not eliminated by natural antibodies (Erickson and Duesberg, 2015)?

But maybe an answer to these questions now exists. In 'What if HPV does NOT cause cervical cancer?',[28] Norma Erickson and Peter H. Duesberg discuss the implications for the virus hypothesis resulting from the findings presented in a paper published in *Molecular Cytogenetics* (2013)[29] of which Peter Duesberg is one of six authors. Erickson and Duesberg suggest that if the findings in this research titled 'Individual karyotypes at the origins of cervical carcinomas' are correct, it is very doubtful that HPV vaccines will protect against cervical cancer (Erickson and Duesberg, 2015).

According to this research, it is not HPV infection that is needed for the development of cervical cancer. Rather, the responsibility lies with 'new abnormal karyotypes'.

Duesberg and co-authors found in their 2013 study that all the cervical cancer cells examined contained "new abnormal karyotypes," a karyotype being "the number, size, and shape of chromosomes in any given organism" (Erickson and Duesberg, 2015). This finding has led the researchers to make the observation that the cervical cancers originated with these karyotypes and not from a virus such as HPV. As Erickson and Duesberg state: "No two cancers are the same" and "All cancers have individual clonal (cells descended from and genetically identical to the parent cell) karyotypes (number, size and shape of chromosomes) and thus phenotypes (expressed physical traits)." But if these cervical cancers were caused by HPV they would be "... more or less the

---

28 <http://sanevax.org/hpv-not-cause-cervical-cancer/>

29 <http://molecularcytogenetics.biomedcentral.com/articles/10.1186/1755-8166-6-44>

same" for they would have had "common transforming proteins" (Erickson and Duesberg, 2015).

The study undertaken by McCormack *et al.* and later discussed by Norma Erickson and one of the authors, Peter Duesberg, builds on the idea that cancer is "a form of speciation," a theory which "proposes that carcinogens initiate carcinogenesis by causing aneuploidy, i.e. losses or gains of chromosomes"(Duesberg *et al.*, 2011). In line with this theory, karyotypic evolutions result in new cancer species which differ from normal cells after exposure to carcinogens such as cigarette smoke or X-rays. Smoking has been implicated in the causation of cervical cancers since the 1970s (McCormack *et al.*, 2013).

Erickson and Duesberg state that the karyotypic speciation theory answers the questions asked about the now entrenched HPV-causes-cancer-hypothesis.

Why would only 1 in 10,000 HPV-infected women develop cervical cancer? (Erickson and Duesberg, 2015).

Erickson and Duesberg suggest that this is because HPV infection and carcinogenesis are two different events. HPV is a very common virus which is typically sexually transmitted at a young age, whereas cancers "originate from a major rearrangement of the karyotypes of normal cells" as seen in their study of cervical cancer cells (McCormack *et al.*, 2013). The fact that this is true for cancers that occur in both HPV-positive and HPV-negative females means "there is no specific correlative evidence that HPV plays any role in causing cervical cancer" (Erickson and Duesberg, 2015). Instead, the 2013 research published in

Molecular Cytogenetics has shown that cervical cancers result from the abnormal karyotypes arising from normal cells.

Why would cervical cancers only develop 20 to 50 years after HPV infection? (Erickson and Duesberg, 2015).

Erickson and Duesberg explain that the huge latent period between HPV infection and carcinogenesis "exclude a direct mechanism of action connecting viral infection and the development of cancer." They state that HPV infection and the development of cancer are two different events. Rather than HPV infection causing cervical cancer, the authors claim that the evidence from the study points to the evolution of "a new cancer-specific karyotype" as causation (2015). This evolution of a new species of abnormal cells — cervical cancer cells — takes time. According to the authors:

> … the chronological discrepancies between HPV infection and carcinogenesis exclude a direct mechanism of action connecting viral infection and the development of cancer. Instead the time-dependent evolution of a new cancer-specific karyotype supports the karyotypic theory of the origin of cervical carcinomas (Erickson and Duesberg, 2015).

Why do cervical carcinomas have individual karyotypes and phenotypes – rather than common phenotypes as predicted by the virus hypothesis? (Erickson and Duesberg, 2015).

There is only a slight chance that cancers caused by this process known as karyotypic speciation will replicate as the same new cancer. Therefore these cancers have individual and occasionally similar phenotypes.

Why are presumably viral cervical carcinomas not immunogenic and thus not eliminated by natural antibodies? (Erickson and Duesberg, 2015).

Karyotypic cancer theory suggests that these cervical carcinomas "are *generated* de novo from cellular chromosomes, genes and proteins", which are not immunogenic (they do not induce an immune response). Therefore they are not eliminated by natural antibodies. If the cancer cells were generated from viral proteins, they would be promptly eradicated by antiviral immunity. According to the authors, the pieces of inactive HPV DNA that can be found in cervical cancers are from infections or warts that occurred 20-50 years before the cancer.

These research findings put a whole new light on the HPV-causes-cervical-cancer hypothesis. And it does answer the above questions that until now have been put conveniently aside.

The Karotypic Speciation Theory of cervical cancer development should not be ignored (Erickson and Duesberg, 2015). However, that is what appears to be happening. When I asked her, what response there had been from the scientific community, Norma Erickson, the co-author of the article replied:

The response from the scientific community has been complete silence. There are a couple of reasons for this. Number one is that if this theory is correct, it blows the whole premise upon which HPV vaccines are manufactured and promoted. It would prove them completely useless except for perhaps preventing genital warts.

The second reason for silence is that it is VERY unpopular to put forth any information that brings current vaccination practices into question.

The silence on this issue speaks volumes. If the theory could be easily discredited, you can bet that those promoting HPV vaccines in particular would have jumped at the opportunity. Since this has not happened, in my mind, this adds credibility to the theory proposed by the 2013 Duesberg *et al.* paper (pers. com., Erickson, 2017).

Conclusion

Journalism can never be silent ...
it must speak, and speak immediately ...

Henry Anatole Grunwald,
former managing editor of *Time Magazine*
(CBC News, 2007)

The story of *Gardasil: Fast-Tracked and Flawed* is a work in progress. We do not yet know the full extent of the damage to the bodies of young girls and boys all around the world after their HPV vaccinations. Nor do we know when, or if, this vaccination program will cease to exist.

As I write these pages, young girls and boys are still lining up to be injected with HPV vaccines without asking any questions. It is high time for a public discussion. What we need are mainstream journalists who are brave enough to tell the stories of sudden death, of permanently damaged girls and boys, and of families in crisis in the wake of Gardasil vaccinations. Only then will politicians who until now endorse, or at least silently condone, the HPV vaccinations of young girls and boys be forced to take a close look at what is happening.

Naomi Fryers is a freelance journalist living in Melbourne. Writing for *Independent Australia* she wants an independent inquiry into whether the public and doctors have been told the truth about Gardasil.

Medical professionals cannot seem to agree on whether Gardasil is safe. Nor can the mainstream media or the legal system. So herein lies the conundrum: where is the moratorium? And at what price comes the prevention of international embarrassment for invested parties? When the truth is so ambiguous that the 'big boys' cannot agree, something is clearly very wrong. It's time for clarity (Fryers, 2016).

Fryers asks her readers not to call her an 'anti-vaxer' for if she had been, she says, then she would not have suffered a severe autoimmune-based neurological reaction after her Gardasil vaccinations (Fryers, 2016). *Independent Australia* is an online progressive journal focusing on politics, democracy, the environment, Australian history and identity. It is not a mainstream newspaper or television station, so sadly lacks the effect that a huge audience could have in challenging the accepted mantra that HPV vaccines are needed to reduce cases of cervical cancer.

In the current media landscape in Australia where the owners of the networks have much say in what makes news, the airing of the problems with Gardasil will be difficult. It needs to be acknowledged that in June 2009 Channel 7's *Sunday Night Program* aired a program about the problems with Gardasil which according to Meryl Dorey from the Australian Vaccination Skeptics-Network (AVN) was a "fairly balanced program" (*Living Wisdom*, 2009). But then this was in 2009 and it is now 2017. In the interim years, the number of people experiencing adverse effects after HPV vaccinations has been growing and there is new research into the effects of aluminium on the brain. Mirza *et al.* have measured the amount of aluminium in the brain tissue from donors who were diagnosed with familial Alzheimer's disease. The levels were found to be extremely high: "… there were values in excess of 10 μg/g [mcg] tissue dry weight in 5 of the 12 individuals" (Mirza *et al.*, 2017, p. 30). The researchers state that the cause of Alzheimer's is not known, but it may be that environmental factors such as aluminium may be revealed as contributing to the disease (Mirza *et al.*, 2017). As has been discussed in *Gardasil: Fast-Tracked and Flawed*, each intramuscular dose of Gardasil contains 225 micrograms of aluminium and studies have shown that these vaccine aluminium adjuvants, used to increase immune response can facilitate the entry of aluminium into the brain (NVIC, 2006).

Research into HPV vaccines is progressing and needs to be part of the public conversation. News that questions the HPV hypothesis also needs to be relayed to the public such as that reported by Thabet *et al.* who found that HPV wasn't the main cause of pre-invasive and invasive cervical cancer among patients in the Delta Region, Egypt. They report the existence of HPV in 39.5% of premalignant lesions and 33.3% in malignant cervical lesions. The researchers suggest that further work is needed in determining the value of HPV vaccinations in their region (Thabet *et al.*, 2014).

Such developments need to be communicated to the public via media stories that bravely explore the aftermath of HPV vaccinations.

Television and radio programs depend on advertising income, as do newspapers. In return they often produce articles and programs that fail to challenge the existing state of affairs. As honorary professor in the School of Humanities and Social Inquiry at the University of Wollongong, Sharon Beder, explains:

> Journalists are free to write what they like if they produce well-written stories 'free of any politically discordant tones', that is, if what they write fits the ideology of those above them in the hierarchy. A story that supports the status quo is generally considered to be neutral and its objectivity is not questioned, while one that challenges the status quo tends to be perceived as having a 'point of view' and therefore biased (Beder, 2004).

Beder writes about the power of corporate advertising and its ability to influence and taper media content so as to attract a certain audience who will succumb to advertising, its considerable influence extending to the editing of content (Beder, 2004). In light of this analysis I am not surprised that the stories of young girls and boys damaged after HPV vaccinations are ignored by mainstream media, or that there has been no attempt to inform the public that as of September 1, 2015, there had been 345 claims filed in the U.S. Federal Vaccine Injury Compensation Program (VICP) for injuries and deaths following HPV vaccination, including 14 deaths and 331 serious injuries (HRSA, Health Resources and Services Administration, 2017). The silence on these deaths and compensation claims is deafening.

Why is there such overwhelming support for the HPV vaccination programs? Perhaps Peter Gøtzsche, the head of the Nordic Cochrane Centre, can help explain. In *Deadly Medicines and Organised Crime: How Big Pharma Has Corrupted Healthcare* (Gøtzsche, 2013), the author compares the activities of the pharmaceutical industry to that of organised crime. The greater part of his book explains how the pharmaceutical industry can manipulate the public. Richard Smith, a former editor of the British Medical Journal (BMJ) and the director of the United Health Group's chronic disease initiative wrote the foreword to the book published on the website of the British Medical Journal (BMJ) titled 'Is the pharmaceutical industry like the mafia?' In his foreword, Smith claims that Gøtzsche is not the first to compare the pharmaceutical industry with organised crime. In his book Gøtzsche quotes a former vice-president of Pfizer:

> It is scary how many similarities there are between this industry and the mob. The mob makes obscene amounts of money, as does this industry. The side effects of organized crime are killings and deaths, and the side effects are the same in this industry. The mob bribes politicians and others, and so does the drug industry (in Gøtzsche, 2013, and quoted by Smith in his Foreword to the book).

Gøtzsche claims that the drug industry has manipulated science "to play up benefits and play down harms of their drugs." He reveals "how the industry has bought doctors, academics, journals, professional and patient organisations, university departments, journalists, regulators, and politicians. These are the methods of the mob" (in Smith, 2013).

Knowing how the system works helps us understand why there is so little reporting of any problems with HPV vaccinations in the mainstream media. But it doesn't excuse the media industry for failing to inform the public that so far HPV vaccines have not prevented a single case of cervical cancer, and that there are thousands of girls and boys who have become ill after vaccination with these medicines. After all, informing the public is their job.

My heart goes out to those girls and boys who have suffered and those still unwell after they were given HPV vaccines. I also extend great sympathy to the parents of these young people, many of whom are experiencing guilt over their consent to HPV vaccination. I urge all those who do experience side effects in Australia to report these reactions to the TGA site,[30] and in the USA to the VAERS[31] website. However, despite there being official sites to record adverse effects, what is being done to follow up these adverse reactions and determine a cause? How can we be sure all adverse effects are recorded? What accountability processes are resulting from these many thousands of recorded adverse events? And importantly, how are the affected young women and men helped to recover from their ill health? The answers to these questions must form part of our activism around ensuring that the story of Gardasil is heard.

As I write this Conclusion to *Gardasil: Fast-Tracked and Flawed*, I am aware we are far from having a satisfactory ending to this upsetting story. It remains to be seen how long it will take for the mainstream media to expose the Gardasil story. In a world where the market in vaccines is worth close to $24 billion and with the staggering prediction that the vaccine market will reach

---

30 Therapeutic Goods Administration: <https://www.tga.gov.au/reporting-problems>

31 VAERS-Vaccine Adverse Event Reporting System: <https://vaers.hhs.gov/index>

an estimated $61 billion in profits by 2020, it is best not to hold your breath (Guzman, 2016).

I believe strongly that we should put the HPV vaccination program on hold. And I suggest that action must also include treatment for those poor girls and boys who have become severely ill after HPV vaccinations — at the expense of the companies reaping millions from these vaccinations, rather than burdening the public purse. As the stories in this book have shown, the injured are often left to suffer for a long time, are misdiagnosed and given inappropriate treatments. If the adverse effects suffered after HPV vaccines were better known to the public and health professionals, then those suffering could be diagnosed swiftly and given treatment. Until the full truth about Gardasil and the other HPV vaccinations is known, and the question about compensation can be asked, I think this is the absolute minimum they deserve. We are well aware of the damage that drugs such as thalidomide caused to unborn babies; the deaths from the arthritis drug Vioxx; from smoking and from asbestos exposure; and as has been presented on these pages, the flaws in this vaccination program. Manufacturers of drugs, vaccines and medical equipment must be accountable.

I hope that this exposé will not only enlighten those who read it, but also inspire them to become active. Actions that we must take include telling this story to friends and family, raising it in public forums and with politicians. And in Australia, we must demand an independent inquiry into the Gardasil story.

Finally I urge readers of *Gardasil: Fast-Tracked and Flawed* to take this important threat to our children's health and wellbeing seriously. What started out as a vaccine fast-tracked to protect against cervical cancer is flawed. Gardasil is a vaccine only effective against a few types of human papilloma virus. Will it ever prevent cervical cancer? We just don't know.

Glossary

AAVP	Asociacion de Afectadas por la Vacuna del Papiloma
ADEM	acute disseminated encephalomyelitis
ADRs	adverse reactions
AIDS	acquired immune deficiency syndrome
AIDWA	All India Democratic Women's Association
AIHW	Australian Institute of Health and Welfare
AVN	Australian Vaccination Skeptics Network
BMJ	British Medical Journal
CDC	Centers for Disease Control and Prevention (USA)
CFDA	China Food and Drug Administration
CIN	cervical intraepithelial neoplasia
CRPS	chronic regional pain syndrome
CSL	Commonwealth Serum Laboratories
DAEN	Database of Adverse Events Notifications (Australia)
DES	Diethylstilbestrol
EMA	European Medicines Agency
FDA	Food and Drug Administration (USA)
FLI	Family Life International
GBS	Guillain-Barré Syndrome
HIV	human immunodeficiency virus
HPV	human papilloma virus
HSV	herpes simplex virus
IARC	International Agency for Research on Cancer
ICMA	Indian Council of Medical Research
IVIG	intravenous immunoglobulin
JSA	Jan Swasthya Abhiyaan
MPL	monophosphoryl lipid A
MRI	magnetic resonance imaging
NIH	National Institutes of Health (USA)
NCI	National Cancer Institute (USA)
NORD	National Organization for Rare Diseases (USA)
NVIC	National Vaccine Information Center (USA)
PATH	Program for Appropriate Technology in Health

PBAC	Pharmaceutical Benefits Advisory Committee (Australia)
PBS	Pharmaceutical Benefits Scheme (Australia)
PET	positron emission topography
POF	premature ovarian failure
POTS	postural orthostatic tachycardia syndrome
PRIA	Public Relations Institute of Australia
REGRET	Reactions and Effects of Gardasil Resulting in Extreme Trauma (Ireland)
RRP	recurrent respiratory papillomatosis
SLE	systemic lupus erythematosus
TGA	Therapeutic Goods Administration (Australia)
VAERS	Vaccine Adverse Events Reporting System (USA)
VCIP	Vaccine Injury Compensation Program
VLP	virus-like particles
WHO	World Health Organisation

Bibliography

Adams, Phillip (2015) 'Why Does Cancer Exist?' *Late Night Live*. ABC. Radio National. December 7; <http://www.abc.net.au/radionational/programs/latenightlive/paul-davies---new-cancer research/6999052>

Agarwal, A K, R Garg, A Ritch and P Sarkar (2007) 'Postural orthostatic tachycardia syndrome'. *Postgraduate Medical Journal*. July, 83(981), pp. 478–480; <https://www.ncbi.nlm.nih.gov/pmc/articles/PMC2600095/>

AIHW (2005) 'Mortality over the twentieth century in Australia: Trends and patterns in major causes of death'. Mortality Surveillance Series No. 4. AIHW Cat. No. PHE73. *Australian Institute of Health and Welfare*, Canberra; <http://www.aihw.gov.au/WorkArea/DownloadAsset.aspx?id=6442459697>

AIHW (2012–13) 'Cervical screening in Australia 2012-13'. *Australian Institute of Health and Welfare*, Canberra; <http://www.aihw.gov.au/WorkArea/DownloadAsset.aspx?id=60129550872>

AIHW (2015) 'Cervical cancer reduced due to screening'. *Australian Institute of Health and Welfare*, Canberra; <http://aihw.gov.au/media-release-detail/?id=60129550866>

AIHW (2016) 'Cervical cancer screening saving lives'. *Australian Institute of Health and Welfare*, Canberra; <http://aihw.gov.au/media-release-detail/?id=60129555150>

Alexandra, Nicole (2014) 'Gardasil: What lack of informed consent did for me?' January 10; <http://sanevax.org/gardasil-lack-informed-consent/>

Alton, Lori (2015) 'FDA approves double the aluminium in new Gardasil vaccine'. *NaturalHealth365*. March 8; <http://www.naturalhealth365.com/gardasil-vaccine-dangers-1341.html>

American Cancer Society (2017) 'Types of Cervical Cancer'; <https://www.cancer.org/cancer/cervical-cancer/about/what-is-cervical-cancer.html>

American College of Pediatricians (2016) 'New Concerns about the Human Papilloma Virus'. January; <https://www.acpeds.org/the-college-speaks/position-statements/health-issues/new-concerns-about-the-human-papillomavirus-vaccine>

The Asahi Shimbun (2013) 'Health ministry withdraws recommendation for cervical cancer vaccine'. *The Asahi Shimbun.* June 15; <https://www.sott.net/article/262825-Japans-health-ministry-withdraws-recommendation-for-cervical-cancer-vaccine>

Beder, Sharon (2004) 'Moulding and Manipulating the News'. *Controversies in Environmental Sociology.* in White, R (ed). Cambridge University Press, Melbourne, pp. 204-220; <http://ro.uow.edu.au/cgi/viewcontent.cgi?article=1043&context=artspapers>

Beran, Ruth (2006) 'Ian Frazer's patent problem'. *Life Scientist.* July 21; <http://www.lifescientist.com.au/content/lab-technology/news/ian-frazers-patent-problem-1263005711>

Bosch, F X, A Lorincz, N Munoz, C Meijer and K V Shah (2002) 'The causal relation between human papillomavirus and cervical cancer'. *Journal of Clinical Pathology.* January 22; <https://www.ncbi.nlm.nih.gov/pmc/articles/PMC1769629/>

Boseley, Sarah (2007) 'Alarm at 'battering ram' tactics over cervical cancer'. *The Guardian.* March 26; <https://www.theguardian.com/society/2007/mar/26/cancercare.health1>

Brenton, Nicholas (2016) 'Acute Disseminated Encephalomyelitis'. December 19; <http://emedicine.medscape.com/article/1147044-overview>

Brogan, Kelly (2015) 'Selling the Fear of Cervical Cancer. The New Gardasil Vaccine: Is It Right for Your Daughter?' *Global Research.* May 15; <http://www.globalresearch.ca/selling-the-fear-of-cervical-cancer-the-new-gardasil-vaccine-is-it-right-for-your-daughter/5449576>

Buncombe, Andrew and Nina Lakhani (2011) 'Without consent: how drugs companies exploit Indian "guinea pigs"'. *Independent.* November 14; <http://www.independent.co.uk/news/world/asia/without-consent-how-drugs-companies-exploit-indian-guinea-pigs-6261919.html>

Californian Legislative information (2015) 'Senate Bill No. 277'. June 30; <https://leginfo.legislature.ca.gov/faces/billNavClient.xhtml?bill_id=201520160SB277>

Cancer Australia (2017a) 'Breast cancer in Australia'; <https://canceraustralia.gov.au/affected-cancer/cancer-types/breast-cancer/breast-cancer-statistics>

Cancer Australia (2017b) 'Bowel cancer': <https://bowel-cancer.canceraustralia.gov.au/statistics>

Cancer Australia (2017c) 'Genetic testing for breast/ovarian cancer risk'; <https://canceraustralia.gov.au/clinical-best-practice/gynaecological-cancers/familial-risk-assessment-fra-boc/genetic-testing>

Cancer Australia (2017d) 'Cervical Cancer in Australia'; <https://cervical-cancer.canceraustralia.gov.au/statistics>

Cancer Council Australia (2013) 'Boys join national HPV vaccination program'. February 15; <http://www.cancer.org.au/news/news-articles/boys-join-national-hpv-vaccination-program.html>

Cancer Council Australia (2016a) 'Cervical Cancer'. June 22; <http://www.cancer.org.au/about-cancer/types-of-cancer/cervical-cancer.html>

Cancer Council Australia (2017) 'Cancer in Australia'. February 9; <http://www.cancer.org.au/about-cancer/what-is-cancer/facts-and-figures.html>

Cancer Council Victoria (2015a) 'Cervical Cancer'. October 1; <http://www.cancervic.org.au/about-cancer/cancer_types/cervical_cancer>

Cancer Council Victoria (2015b) 'Treatment for Cervical Council'. October 1; <http://www.cancervic.org.au/aboutcancer/cancer_types/cervical_cancer/treatment_for_cervical_cancer.html>

Capilla, Alicia (2015) 'Spain: AAVP responds to EMA conclusion on HPV vaccine safety'. November 6; <http://sanevax.org/spain-aavp-responds-to-ema-conclusion-on-hpv-vaccine-safety/>

CBC News (2007) 'Best. Journalism Quotes. Ever'. July 3; <http://www.cbsnews.com/news/best-journalism-quotes-ever/>

CDC (2014) 'Eileen's Cancer Survivor Story'. *Centers for Disease Control and Prevention*; <https://www.cdc.gov/cancer/knowledge/survivor_stories/eileen.htm>

CDC (2015) 'Vaccine Adjuvants'. *Centers for Disease Control and Prevention.* August 28; <www.cdc.gov/vaccinesafety/>

CDC (2016) 'How Many Cancers Are Linked with HPV Each Year?' *Centers for Disease Control and Prevention.* July 6; <https://www.cdc.gov/cancer/hpv/statistics/cases.htm#5>

Chin, Richard (2016) 'Surrogate Endpoints'. *Clinicaltrialist;.* <https://clinicaltrialist.wordpress.com/clinical/surrogate-endpoints/>

Chomet, Jane and Julian Chomet (1989) *Cervical Cancer: All you and your partner need to know about its prevention, detection and treatment.* Grapevine, London.

Clulow, Kristin (2012) 'My Personal Gardasil Journey'. July 9; <http://sanevax.org/my-personal-gardasil-journey/>

Clulow, Kristin (2013) 'They thought I'd had a stroke'; <https://helenlobato.com/2013/08/24/they-thought-id-had-a-stroke/#comments>

Clulow, Kristin (2014) 'My Road to Recovery Post-Gardasil'. May 14; <http://sanevax.org/road-recovery-post-gardasil/>

Cochrane Nordic (2017) 'About us'. *Cochrane*; <http://nordic.cochrane.org/about-us>

Coleman, Michael (2013) 'War on cancer and the influence of the medical-industrial complex'. *Journal of Cancer Policy*. June 17; <http://www.journalcancerpolicy.net/article/S2213-5383(13)00007-6/pdf>

Colvin, Mark (2007) 'Cervical cancer vaccination program begins'. *ABC*. April 2; <http://www.abc.net.au/pm/content/2007/s1887834.htm>

Conis, Elena (2014) *Vaccine Nation: America's Changing Relationship with Immunization*. The University of Chicago Press, Chicago.

CSL (2016) 'Gardasil'. <http://www.csl.com.au/s1/cs/auhq/1196562765747/Web_Product_C/1196562633137/ProductDetail.htm>

Cuomo, Margaret (2012) 'Are We Wasting Billions Seeking a Cure for Cancer?' *The Daily Beast*. February 10; <http://www.thedailybeast.com/articles/2012/10/02/are-we-wasting-billions-seeking-a-cure-for-cancer.html>

Dana-Farber Cancer Institute (2013) 'The War on Cancer, 40 years later'. Dana-Farber Cancer Institute. November 21; <http://blog.dana-farber.org/insight/2011/12/the-war-on-cancer-40-years-later/>

Davies, Paul (2012) 'Cancer can teach us about our own evolution'. *The Guardian*. November 19; <https://www.theguardian.com/commentisfree/2012/nov/18/cancer-evolution-bygone-biological-age>

Dayton, Leigh (1997) 'Cervical Cancer Vaccine Getting Closer'. *Sydney Morning Herald*. Nov 13.

Department of Health (2009) 'Chief Medical Officer Guidance on revaccination where HPV vaccine doses have been given at less than recommended minimum intervals'. January; <http://www.immunise.health.gov.au/internet/immunise/publishing.nsf/Content/cmo-full-advice-hpv-cnt>

Department of Health (2015) 'National Cervical Screening Program'. May 10; <http://www.cancerscreening.gov.au/internet/screening/publishing.nsf/Content/future-changes-cervical>

DES Action (2016) 'Clear Cell Adenocarcinoma (CCA) of the Vagina and Cervix'. <http://www.desaction.org/des-daughters/>

The *Dijene* HPV Test (2017) 'HPV Vaccination FAQS'; <http://www.thehpvtest.com/about-hpv/hpv-vaccine-faqs/>

Dorey, Meryl (2009) 'Channel 7 Sunday Night Program – A Show About the Dangers of Gardasil Vaccine'. *Living Wisdom.* June; <http://archive.constantcontact.com/fs082/1101800214009/archive/1102624430875.html>

Dorey, Meryl (2016) 'Vaccination Schedules in Australia'. *Australian Vaccination-skeptics Network Inc.* February 23; <https://avn.org.au/vaccination-information/general-vaccination-information/>

Doyle, Arthur Conan (1928) *The Adventures of Sherlock Holmes.* MBI Publishing Company, Minneapolis.

Duesberg, Peter H and Jody R Schwartz (1992). 'Latent Viruses and Mutated Oncogenes: No Evidence for Pathogenicity'. *Duesberg on Aids*; <http://www.duesberg.com/papers/ch5.html>

Duesberg, Peter (1996) *Inventing the Aids Virus.* Regnery Publishing Inc., Washington.

Duesberg Peter, Daniele Mandrioli, Amanda McCormack and Joshua M. Nicholson (2011) 'Is carcinogenesis a form of speciation?' *Cell Cycle* Vol. 10, Issue 13, July 1; <http://www.tandfonline.com/doi/abs/10.4161/cc.10.13.16352>

Dyson, Linda (1986) *Cervical Cancer: A book for every woman.* Nelson. Melbourne.

Erickson, Norma (2010) 'Gardasil Approval: FDA Apparently Does Not Follow Its Own Rules'. December 12; <http://sanevax.org/gardasil-approval-fda-apparently-does-not-follow-its-own-rules/>

Erickson, Norma (2014a) 'France: Meeting to debate HPV vaccines, Gardasil and Cervarix'. June 25; <http://sanevax.org/france-meeting-debate-hpv-vaccines-gardasil-cervarix/>

Erickson, Norma (2014b) 'Gardasil: Criminal complaint filed in Spain'. August 2; <http://sanevax.org/gardasil-criminal-complaint-filed-spain/>

Erickson, Norma (2014c) 'FDA approved Gardasil 9: Malfeasance or Stupidity?' December 17; <http://sanevax.org/fda-approved-gardasil-9-malfeasance-or-stupidity/>

Erickson, Norma (2015) 'Vaccines: The Battle for Informed Consent'. May 30; <http://sanevax.org/vaccines-the-battle-for-informed-consent/>

Erickson, Norma and Peter Duesberg (2015) 'What if HPV does NOT cause cervical cancer?' January 20; <http://sanevax.org/hpv-not-cause-cervical-cancer/>

Erickson, Norma (2016a) 'HPV Vaccines Vaers Reports to March 2016'; <http://sanevax.org>

Erickson, Norma (2016b) 'Dr. Sin Hang Lee recommends China postpone HPV vaccinations'. August 22; <http://sanevax.org/dr-lee-recommends-china-postpone-hpv-vaccinations/>

Erickson, Norma (2017) 'Re: What if HPV does NOT cause cervical cancer?' personal communication with Helen Lobato, January 10.

Fanning, Ellen (2011) '60 Minutes Australia'. *Channel 9.* June 10; <https://www.youtube.com/watch?v=u0lsz86WBLk>

Field, Scott S (2016) 'New Concerns about the Human Papillomavirus Vaccine'. *American College of Pediatricians.* January 16; <http://www.acpeds.org/the-college-speaks/position-statements/health-issues/new-concerns-about-the-human-papillomavirus-vaccine>

Fifield, Anna (2015) 'The science doesn't support them, but Japanese anti-vaxxers are winning on HPV'. *The Washington Post.* November 10; <https://www.washingtonpost.com/news/worldviews/wp/2015/11/10/the-science-doesnt-support-it-but-japanese-anti-vaxxers-are-winning-on-hpv/>

Fisher, Barbara Loe, (2008) 'Examining the Science and Politics of HPV Vaccine'. *Vaccine Awakening.* May 9; <http://vaccineawakening.blogspot.com.au/2008/05/examining-science-politics-of-hpv.html>

Fisher, Barbara Loe (2009a) 'Preventing Gardasil Vaccine Injuries and Deaths'. *National Vaccine Information Centre.* July 14; <http://www.nvic.org/NVIC-Vaccine-News/July-2009/Preventing-Gardasil-Vaccine-Injuries-Deaths.aspx>

Fisher, Barbara Loe (2009b) 'Gardasil Death and Brain Damage: A National Tragedy'. *National Vaccine Information Center.* September 2; <http://www.nvic.org/NVIC-Vaccine-News/February-2009/Monday,-February-09,-2009-Gardasil-Death---Brain-D.aspx>

Fisher, Barbara Loe (2010) 'HPV Vaccine: The Lethal Medical Failure That's Still Recommended by Your Doctor'. December 29; <http://articles.mercola.com/sites/articles/archive/2010/12/29/why-india-has-stopped-giving-hpv-vaccines.aspx>

Fisher, Barbara Loe (2016) 'Human Papillomavirus (HPV)'. *National Vaccine Information Center*; <http://www.nvic.org/Vaccines-and-Diseases/hpv.aspx>

FLI Australia (2013) 'Truth and Gardasil: Interview with Dr Deirdre Little'. *Family Life International*. April 24; <https://www.youtube.com/watch?v=TBs6BD-Ec44>

Fox, Michaela (2015) 'The heartbreak or relief of hysterectomies'. *news.com.au*. July 15; <http://www.news.com.au/lifestyle/health/health-problems/the-heartbreak-or-relief-of-hysterectomies/news-story/4ad9fd7d6bef24c9710e5041c9dfa979>

Fryers, Naomi (2016) 'Gardasil a gift for potential cancers patients or a prick that can maim'. *Independent Australia*. April 10; <https://independentaustralia.net/life/life-display/gardasil-a-gift-for-potential-cancer-patients-or-a-prick-that-can-maim,8865>

Gardasil Commercial (2006) 'One Less'. Youtube; <https://www.youtube.com/watch?v=hJ8x3KR75fA>

Gillaspy, Rebecca (2017) 'What are Cytokines? – Definition, Types and Function'; <http://study.com/academy/lesson/what-are-cytokines-definition-types-function.html>

Gøtzsche, Peter, C (2013) *Deadly Medicines and Organised Crime: How Big Pharma Has Corrupted Healthcare*. Taylor and Francis Ltd, London.

Gøtzsche, Peter, C (2016) 'Complaint to the European Medicines Agency (EMA) over maladministration at the EMA'. May 26; <http://nordic.cochrane.org/sites/nordic.cochrane.org/files/uploads/ResearchHighlights/Complaint-to-EMA-over-EMA.pdf>

Green, Gertrude and Renate Klein (2008) 'About'. *Gardasil: Women Hurt by Medicine;* <https://womenhurtbymedicine.wordpress.com/about-this-site/>

Green, Gertrude (2009) 'Jessica's Story'. *Gardasil: Women Hurt By Medicine*. August 31; <https://womenhurtbymedicine.wordpress.com/page/2/>

Greer, Germaine (1999) *The Whole Woman*. Doubleday, London.

GSK (2007) 'Cervarix® Product Information'. *GlaxoSmithKline*; <http://www.gsk.com.au/resources.ashx/vaccineproductschilddataproinfo/89/FileName/87DBF733088C2D2DD29382F0255BC726/PI_Cervarix.pdf>

GSK (2016) 'GSK announces Cervarix™ approved in China to help protect women from cervical cancer'. *GlaxoSmithKline*. July 18; <https://www.gsk-china.com/en-gb/media/press-releases/2016/gsk-announces-cervarix-approved-in-china-to-help-protect-women-from-cervical-cancer/>

The Guardian (2015) 'Older women ignoring cervical cancer danger'. June 15; <https://www.theguardian.com/society/2015/jun/15/older-women-ignoring-cervical-cancer-danger>

Gucciardi, Anthony (2011) 'Gardasil Victims Take Legal Action Against Merck Over Miscarriage, Deadly Reactions'. *Activist Post*. November 10; <http://www.activistpost.com/2011/11/gardasil-victims-take-legal-action.html>

Guzman, Timothy (2016) 'New Report says "Vaccine Market" Worth $61 Billion by 2020'. *Global Research*. January 26; <http://www.globalresearch.ca/big-pharma-and-big-profits-the-multibillion-dollar-vaccine-market/5503945>

Harris, Ian (2016) *Surgery, The Ultimate Placebo*. New South Publishing, Sydney.

Hart, Elizabeth (2013) 'Gardasil: Australia takes the lead, the story behind the headlines'. May 1; < http://sanevax.org/gardasil-australia-takes-the-lead/>

Health Impact News (2014) 'Merck's Former Doctor Predicts that Gardasil will become the Greatest Medical Scandal of All Time'. April 15; <http://healthimpactnews.com/2014/mercks-former-doctor-predicts-that-gardasil-will-become-the-greatest-medical-scandal-of-all-time/>

Heitmann, Erica and Diane Harper (2012) '2 3 Prophylactic HPV Vaccines and Prevention of Cervical Intraepithelial Neoplasia'. in *Current Obstetrics and Gynaecology* 1(3), September; <https://www.researchgate.net/publication/229540730_2_3_Prophylactic_HPV_Vaccines_and_Prevention_of_Cervical_Intraepithelial_Neoplasia>

HRSA (2017) 'National Vaccine Injury Compensation Program'. *Health Resources and Services Administration*, U.S. Department of Health and Human Services; <https://www.hrsa.gov/vaccinecompensation/data/vicpmonthlyreporttemplate3_1_17.pdf>

HSE Immunisation (2017) 'HPV Vaccine Safety'; <http://www.hse.ie/eng/health/Immunisation/pubinfo/schoolprog/HPV/hpvvaccinesafety/>

Illich, Ivan (1976) *Medical Nemesis: The Expropriation of Health.* Pantheon Books, New York.

Incao, Phillip (2006) 'How Vaccinations Work'; <http://www.whale.to/vaccine/incao.html>

International Agency for Research on Cancer (1989) *Human Papillomavirus and Cervical Cancer.* IARC Publication No. 94; <https://www.iarc.fr/en/publications/books/iarc50/IARC_Ch4.2.5_web.pdf>

International Agency for Research on Cancer (1995) 'Human Papillomaviruses HPV'; <http://www.inchem.org/documents/iarc/vol64/hpv.html>

International Agency for Research on Cancer (2005) 'Use of screening for cervical cancer'. Chapter 3 in *IARC Handbooks of Cancer Prevention.* Volume 10.; <https://www.iarc.fr/en/publications/pdfs-online/prev/handbook10/handbook10-chap3.pdf>

Jana (2016) 'Cervarix: New medical conditions for both my daughters'. April 30; <http://sanevax.org/cervarix-new-medical-conditions-daughters/>

Jasmine (2017) 'Jasmine – Gardasil Experience'. Email Correspondence with Helen Lobato. March 3.

Jenny (2016) 'Gardasil: No benefit for us!' February 10; <http://sanevax.org/gardasil-no-benefit-for-us/>

Jensen, Kirsten E, Sven Schmiedel, Bodil Norrild, Kirsten Frederiksen, Thomas Iftner and Susanne K. Kjaer (2012) 'Parity as a cofactor for high-grade cervical disease among women with persistent human papillomavirus infection: a 13-year follow-up'. *British Journal of Medicine.* November 20; <http://www.nature.com/bjc/journal/v108/n1/full/bjc2012513a.html>

Jiji (2016) 'Lawsuit over cervical cancer vaccines to drag on as health ministry fights on'. *The Japan Times.* October 24; <http://www.japantimes.co.jp/news/2016/10/24/national/crime-legal/lawsuit-cervical-cancer-vaccines-drag-health-ministry-fights/#.WLi9srycONI>

Kent, Christine (2012) 'The Role of Glycogen in Vulvovaginal Health'. *Whole Woman Inc.* <https://wholewoman.com/blog/?p=1041>

King, Madonna (2013) *Ian Frazer: The man who saved a million lives.* University of Queensland Press, Brisbane.

Klein, Renate and Melinda Tankard Reist (2007) 'Gardasil: We must not ignore the risks'. *On Line Opinion*. June 1; <http://www.onlineopinion.com.au/view.asp?article=5917&page=0>

Klein, Renate (2008) 'The Gardasil miracle coming undone?' *On Line Opinion*. August 21; <http://www.onlineopinion.com.au/view.asp?article=7786&page=0>

Klein, Renate and Helen Lobato (2013) 'Australia must also caution on Gardasil'. *On Line Opinion*. June 28; <http://www.onlineopinion.com.au/view.asp?article=15181>

La Vigne, Patrice (2015) 'European Agency Declares HPV Vaccines Safe, But Denmark, Japan Skeptical'. *The Vaccine Reaction*. December 4; <http://www.thevaccinereaction.org/2015/12/european-agency-declares-hpv-vaccines-safe-but-denmark-japan-skeptical/>

Lee, Sin Hang (2015) 'Expert Report in the Matter of Gomez v. United States Department of Health'. November; <http://sanevax.org/wp-content/uploads/2015/11/Gomez-v-USDOH-expert-report.pdf>

Little, Deirdre, Therese and Harvey Rodrick Grenville Ward (2012) *BMJ Case Reports* 'Premature ovarian failure 3 years after menarche in a 16-year-old girl following human papillomavirus vaccination'; <http://search.proquest.com.ezproxy.slv.vic.gov.au/docview/1783067165/3228694EACB94A1FPQ/1?accountid=13905>

Lobato, Helen (2005) 'The Politics of Pap Smears'. *New Matilda*. November 22; <https://newmatilda.com/2005/11/22/politics-pap-smears/>

Lobato, Helen (2007) 'Thanks Tony Abbott'. *Inform Yourself*; <http://www.informyourself.com.au/abbott.html>

Lobato, Helen (2014) 'A new HPV vaccine is approved amid global concerns over Gardasil'. December 28; <https://helenlobato.com/2014/12/28/a-new-hpv-vaccine-is-approved-amid-global-concerns-over-gardasil/>

Lobato, Helen (2015) 'What's wrong with the new HPV test?' October 8; <http://helenlobato.com/2015/10/08/whats-wrong-with-the-new-hpv-test/>

Löwy, Llana (2011) *A Woman's Disease: The history of cervical cancer*. Oxford University Press, Oxford.

Macat (2016) '50 of the most profound quotes you'll ever read'. March 17; <https://www.macat.com/blog/profound-quotes/>

Macmillan (2015) 'What Is Cervical Intra-Epithelial Neoplasia (Cin)?' *Macmillan.* May 31; <http://www.macmillan.org.uk/information-and-support/diagnosing/causes-and-risk-factors/pre-cancerous-conditions/cin.html>

Mandal, Ananya (2014) 'Cancer History'. *News Medical.* February 21; <http://www.news-medical.net/health/Cancer-History.aspx>

Mayo Clinic (2016) 'Cervical Dysplasia: Is it Cancer?'; <http://www.mayoclinic.org/diseases-conditions/cervical-cancer/expert-answers/cervical-dysplasia/faq-20058142>

McColl, Gina (2007) 'Healthcare's Sticking Point'. *The Age.* February 25; <http://www.theage.com.au/news/national/healthcares-sticking-point/2007/02/24/1171734074136.html?page=fullpage#contentSwap2>

McCormack, Amanda, Jiang Lan Fan, Max Duesberg, Matthew Bloomfield, Christian Fiala and Peter Duesberg (2013) 'Individual karyotypes at the origins of cervical carcinomas'. *Molecular Cytogenetics.* October 17; <http://molecularcytogenetics.biomedcentral.com/articles/10.1186/1755-8166-6-44>

McIntyre, Peter (2005) 'Finding the viral link: the story of Harald zur Hausen'. *Cancerworld.* July-August; <http://www.cancerworld.org/pdf/6737_cw7_32_37_Masterpiece%20(2).pdf>

Merck (2011) 'Highlights of Prescribing Information'; <https://www.merck.com/product/usa/pi_circulars/g/gardasil/gardasil_pi.pdf>

Merck (2016) 'Patient Information about GARDASIL® 9'. <https://www.merck.com/product/usa/pi_circulars/g/gardasil_9/gardasil_9_ppi.pdf>

Mercola, Joseph (2011) 'Aluminum: The Neurotoxin Far Worse than Mercury ...' September 21; <http://articles.mercola.com/sites/articles/archive/2011/09/21/could-this-be-the-most-dangerous-aspect-of-vaccines.aspx>

Mercola, Joseph (2012) 'Are You Concerned Over Genetically Modified Vaccines?'; <http://articles.mercola.com/sites/articles/archive/2012/10/02/vicky-debold-on-gmo-vaccines.aspx>

Mirza, Ambreen, Andrew King, Claire Troakes and Christopher Exley (2016) 'Aluminium in brain tissue in familial Alzheimer's disease'. *Journal of Trace Elements in Medicine and Biology.* pp. 30-36. March, 2017; <http://www.sciencedirect.com/science/article/pii/S0946672X16303777>

Mulcahy, Nick (2016) 'GSK's HPV Vaccine, Cervarix, No Longer Available in US'. October 24; <http://www.medscape.com/viewarticle/870853>

Muñoz, N, F X Bosch and O M Jensen (Eds) (1989) *Human Papillomavirus and Cervical Cancer. IARC Publications* No. 94; <https://www.iarc.fr/en/publications/books/iarc50/IARC_Ch4.2.5_web.pdf>

National Cervical Cancer Coalition (2016) 'Cervical Cancer Overview'; <http://www.nccc-online.org/hpvcervical-cancer/cervical-cancer-overview/>

NCI (2011). 'Diethylstilbestrol (DES) and Cancer'. National Cancer Institute. October 5; <http://www.cancer.gov/about-cancer/causes-prevention/risk/hormones/des-fact-sheet>

NIH (2013) 'Cervical Cancer.' National Institutes of Health. March 29; <https://report.nih.gov/nihfactsheets/viewfactsheet.aspx?csid=76>

NIH (2017) 'Complex Regional Pain Syndrome Fact Sheet'. National Institute of Neurological Disorders and Stroke. January; <https://www.ninds.nih.gov/Disorders/Patient-Caregiver-Education/Fact-Sheets/Complex-Regional-Pain-Syndrome-Fact-Sheet>

Nobel Prize (2008) 'The Nobel Prize in Physiology or Medicine 2008'; <http://www.nobelprize.org/nobel_prizes/medicine/laureates/2008/>

NORD (2016) 'Recurrent Respiratory Papillomatosis'. National Organisation for Rare Disorders; <https://rarediseases.org/rare-diseases/recurrent-respiratory-papillomatosis/>

NVIC (2006) 'Mercks's Gardasil Vaccine Not Proven Safe for Little Girls'. National Vaccine Information Center. June 27; <http://www.nvic.org/nvic-archives/pressrelease/gardasilgirls.aspx>

NVIC (2007) 'Gardasil and HPV Infection'. National Vaccine Information Center. February 21; <http://www.nvic.org/nvic-archives/pressrelease/hpvfeb212007.aspx>

NVIC (2016) 'Human Papilloma Virus'. National Vaccine Information Center; <http://www.nvic.org/Vaccines-and-Diseases/HPV.aspx>

NVIC (2017) 'Medalert'. National Vaccine Information Center; <http://www.medalerts.org/vaersdb/findfield.php?EVENTS=on&PAGENO=12&PERPAGE=10&ESORT=&REVERSESORT=&SEX=Male&VAX=(HPV2+HPV4+HPV9+HPVX)&VAXTYPES=(HPV)>

NVIC (2017b) 'Frequently Asked Questions About Vaccine Reactions'. National Vaccine Information Center; <http://www.nvic.org/faqs/vaccine-reactions.aspx>

Off The Radar (2016) 'Gardasil Ingredients'; <http://www.offtheradar.co.nz/vaccines/52-gardasil-ingredients.html>

Otake, Tomoko (2016) 'Cervical cancer vaccine suit filed over side effects'. *The Japan Times*. July 27; <http://www.japantimes.co.jp/news/2016/07/27/national/crime-legal/cervical-cancer-vaccine-suit-filed-over-side-effects/#. WLjAP7ycONI>

Pandey, Vineeta (2010) 'Cancer Vaccine Programme Suspended After 4 Girls Die'. *DNA*. April 8; <http://www.dnaindia.com/node/1368681%3E>

Paras, Tara (2016) 'Flashback: Japan withdraws support for controversial HPV vaccines'. *NEWSTARGET*. November 23; <http://www.newstarget. com/2016-11-23-flashback-japan-withdrawls-support-for-controversial-hpv-vaccines.html>

Parker-Hope, Tara (2008) 'Blaming the Media for Gardasil Hype'. *New York Times*. August 29; <http://well.blogs.nytimes.com/2008/08/29/blaming-the-media-for-gardasil-hype/?_r=0>

Parkin D Max, Freddie Bray, J Ferlay, and Paola Pisani (2005) 'Global Cancer Statistics, 2002'. *CA: A Cancer Journal for Clinicians*. Issue 55; <http://www. ph.ucla.edu/epi/faculty/zhang/courses/epi242/f08/week03/reading%20 week%203-1a.pdf >

PATH (2017) 'Leading innovation in global health'; <http://www.path.org/about/>

PBS (2016) 'Pharmaceutical Benefits Advisory Committee (PBAC) Membership'. Department of Health; <http://www.pbs.gov.au/info/industry/listing/participants/pbac>

Perunovic, Branko (2013) 'Cervix Carcinoma Clear cell carcinoma (adenocarcinoma)'; <http://www.pathologyoutlines.com/topic/cervixclearcell.html>

Piper-Terry, Marcella (2016) 'Gardasil HPV Vaccine Trial Using Infants as Young as One Year of Age'. *Vaccine Impact*. May 10; <http://vaccineimpact. com/2016/gardasil-hpv-vaccine-trial-using-infants-as-young-as-one-year-of-age/>

Pitt, Jolie, A (2015) 'Angelina Jolie Pitt: Diary of a Surgery'. *New York Times*. March 24; <http://www.nytimes.com/2015/03/24/opinion/angelina-jolie-pitt-diary-of-a-surgery.html?_r=0>

Public Relations Institute Australia (2007) 'PRIA Golden Target Awards GARDASIL Finalist Entry 30 July; <http://www.pria.com.au/documents/item/6238>

Quilliam, Susan (1989) *Positive Smear*. Penguin Books, London.

Renter, Elizabeth (2013) 'Developer of HPV Vaccines Blasts the Vaccines for Dangers, False Claims'. *Natural Society*. August 31; <http://naturalsociety.com/hpv-vaccine-developer-blasts-vaccines-dangers-false-claims/>

Roberts, Janine (2008) *Fear of the Invisible: How Scared Should We Be of Viruses and Vaccines, HIV and Aids.* Impact, Bristol.

Roberts, Janine (2009) 'HPV Vaccine Mysteries: Why is a Nobel Award being given for this on December 10th?' *Vaccine Choice Canada*. January 20; <http://vaccinechoicecanada.com/wp-content/documents/VRAN-HPV-Vaccine-Mysteries-by-Janine-Roberts.pdf>

Sama: Resource Group for Women and Health (2010a) 'Press Conference on HPV Vaccines'. April 8; <https://samawomenshealth.wordpress.com/2010/04/>

Sama: Resource Group for Women and Health (2010b) 'Trial and Error: Ethical Violations of HPV Vaccination Trials in India'. May 17; <https://samawomenshealth.wordpress.com/2010/05/>

SaneVax (2013) 'India: HPV vaccines Gardasil and Cervarix make it to the Supreme Court'. January 16; <http://sanevax.org/india-hpv-vaccines-gardasil-and-cervarix-make-it-to-the-supreme-court/>

SaneVax (2017a) 'Welcome to SaneVax'; <http://sanevax.org>

SaneVax (2017b) 'HPV Vaccine Vaers Reports to March 2017'; <http://sanevax.org>

Sarojini N B, Sandhya Srinivasan, Y Madhavi, S Srinivasan and Anjali Shenoi (2010a) 'The HPV Vaccine: Science, Ethics and Regulation'; <http://ciperchile.cl/wp-content/uploads/Papiloma_HPV_Vaccine-INDIA-TRIALS.pdf>

Schmidt, Emma (2011) 'Woman drops legal action against makers of Gardasil'. *Waverley Leader*. November 29; <http://search.proquest.com.ezproxy.slv.vic.gov.au/anznews/docview/906518970/717C2B501D0945AEPQ/1?accountid=13905>

Scott, J (1990) 'Dangerous Liasions.' *Los Angeles Times Magazine*. March 11; <http://articles.latimes.com/1990-03-11/magazine/tm-9_1_sexually-transmitted-disease>

Sharav, Vera (2007) 'HPV Vaccine Researcher Blasts Mandatory Marketing'. *Alliance for Human Research Protection*. March 13; <http://ahrp.org/hpv-vaccine-researcher-blasts-mandatory-marketing/>

Shepard, Elizabeth. M (2011) 'George Papanicolaou: Development of the Pap Smear'. Weill Cornell Medicine. June 29; <http://library.weill.cornell.edu/george-papanicolaou-development-pap-smear>

Shulman. Alix, Kates (1996) *Read Emma Speaks: An Emma Goldman Reader*. Third Edition. Open Road Integrated Media, New York.

Sifferlin, Alexandra (2014) 'FDA Approves First HPV Test For Primary Cervical Cancer Screening'. TIME Health. *April 25*; <http://time.com/76352/fda-cervical-cancer-screening/>

Sikora, Karol (2009) 'At last we're talking about the Big C: Cancer specialist says we can all learn from Jade Goody'. *Daily Mail Australia*. February 22; <http://www.dailymail.co.uk/debate/article-1151900/PROFESSOR-KAROL-SIKORA-At-talking-Big-C---What-learn-Jade-Goody.html#ixzz3uSgdyga3>

Smith, Emma (2014) 'HPV: the whole story, warts and all'. *Cancer Research UK*. September 16; <http://scienceblog.cancerresearchuk.org/2014/09/16/hpv-the-whole-story-warts-and-all/>

Smith, Richard (2013) 'Is the pharmaceutical industry like the mafia?' *The British Medical Journal*. September 10; <http://blogs.bmj.com/bmj/2013/09/10/richard-smith-is-the-pharmaceutical-industry-like-the-mafia/>

Stevens, Matthew (2006) 'Howard rescues Gardasil from Abbott poison pill'. *The Australian*. November 11; <http://www.theaustralian.com.au/archive/business/howard-rescues-gardasil-from-abbott-poison-pill/story-e6frg9lx-1111112503504>

Strom, Marcus (2015) 'Cancer theorist Paul Davies to speak on the disease's evolutionary history'. *The Sydney Morning Herald*. December 2; <http://www.smh.com.au/national/health/controversial-cancer-theorist-paul-davies-to-speak-on-the-diseases-evolutionary-history-20151124-gl6l0d.html>

Sydney Morning Herald (2006) 'Gardasil Fact'. November 29; <http://www.smh.com.au/news/national/gardasil-facts/2006/11/29/1164476257853.html>

Thabet, Mahmoud, Reda Hemida, Mohammad Hasan, Maged Elshamy, Mohammad Elfaraash and Mohammad Emam (2014) 'Human papillomavirus (HPV) is not the main cause of preinvasive and invasive cervical cancer among patients in Delta Region, Egypt'. <https://www.researchgate.net/publication/269714287_Human_papillomavirus_HPV_is_not_the_main_cause_of_preinvasive_and_invasive_cervical_cancer_among_patients_in_Delta_Region_Egypt>

Therapeutic Goods Administration (2015) 'Gardasil (quadrivalent human papillomavirus vaccine) update 2'. Department of Health May 13; <https://www.tga.gov.au/alert/gardasil-quadrivalent-human-papillomavirus-vaccine-update-2>

Therapeutic Goods Administration (2017) 'Database of Adverse Event Notifications – medicines'. Department of Health; <http://apps.tga.gov.au/PROD/DAEN/daen-report.aspx>

Tomljenovic, Lucija and Christopher Shaw (2012) 'Death after Quadrivalent Human Papilloma Virus (HPV) Vaccination: Causal or Coincidental?' *Pharmaceutical Regulatory Affairs: Open Access.* October 4; <http://www.rescuepost.com/files/ltshaw-death-after-quadrivalent-hpv-vaccination-pharma-reg-affairs-2012.pdf>

Tomljenovic, Lucija (2015) 'Forced Vaccinations: For the Greater Good?' *Vaccine Choice Canada.* Spring edition; <http://vaccinechoicecanada.com/wp-content/uploads/Forced-Vaccinations-For-the-Greater-Good-Tomljenovic.pdf>

Tunley, Stephen (2011) 'Stephen Tunley Writes to *60 Minutes*'. August 14; <http://sanevax.org/steven-tunley-writes-to-60-minutes/>

Tunley, Stephen (2016) 'Your letter to '60' minutes'. Email correspondence with Helen Lobato. June 6.

TV3 Ireland (2016) 'Gardasil Girls in Ireland'. *The Vaccine Reaction.* January 10; <http://www.thevaccinereaction.org/2016/01/gardasil-girls-in-ireland-tv3-hpv-documentary/>

The University of Queensland (2017) 'Professor Ian Frazer AC, FRS, FAA'; <http://www.di.uq.edu.au/professor-ian-frazer>

Uniquest (2014) 'From Idea to Impact'. The University of Queensland; <http://uniquest.com.au>

Uniquest (2016) 'Gardasil: A Global Solution to Reducing Cervical Cancer'. *The University of Queensland*; <http://uniquest.com.au/filething/get/8631/Gardasil%20Commercialisation%20Story.pdf>

Uppsala Monitoring Centre (2017) (UMC) 'About us'. Uppsala Monitoring Centre; <https://www.who-umc.org/#>

U.S. Food and Drug Administration (2006) 'Gardasil (Human Papillomavirus Vaccine) Questions and Answers'. FDA. June 8; <http://www.fda.gov/BiologicsBloodVaccines/Vaccines/QuestionsaboutVaccines/ucm096052.htm>

U.S. Food and Drug Administration (2014b) 'FDA approves Gardasil 9 for prevention of certain cancers caused by five additional types of HPV'. FDA. December 10; <http://www.fda.gov/NewsEvents/Newsroom/PressAnnouncements/ucm426485.htm>

U.S. National Institutes of health (2013) '4-valent HPV Vaccine to Treat Recurrent Respiratory Papillomatosis in Children'. <https://clinicaltrials.gov/ct2/show/record/NCT01995721>

Vn, Sreeja (2013) 'India Government-Appointed Panel Accuses U.S.-Based Non-Profit Group, PATH, Of Violating Clinical Trial Norms During Its Cervical Cancer Study On Children, Women'. *International Business Times.* April 9; <http://www.ibtimes.com/india-government-appointed-panel-accuses-us-based-non-profit-group-path-violating-1402530>

Wang, Sophia S, Rosemary E Zuna, Nicholas Wentzensen, S Terence Dunn, Mark E Sherman, Michael A Gold, Mark Schiffman, Sholom Wacholder, Richard A Allen, Ingrid Block, Kim Downing, Jose Jeronimo, J Daniel Carreon, Mahboobeh Safaeian, David Brown and Joan L, Walker (2009) 'Human papillomavirus (HPV) cofactors by disease progression and HPV types in the Study to Understand Cervical Cancer Early Endpoints and Determinants (SUCCEED)'. *Cancer, Epidemiology, Biomarkers and Prevention.* January; <https://www.ncbi.nlm.nih.gov/pmc/articles/PMC2952430/>

WebMD (2017) 'Cervical Dysplasia'; <http://www.webmd.com/cancer/cervical-cancer/cervical-dysplasia-symptoms-causes-treatments#1>

WHO (2007) 'Human papillomavirus and HPV vaccines: a review'. *Bulletin of the World Health Organisation.* September; <http://www.who.int/bulletin/volumes/85/9/06-038414/en/>

WHO (2008) 'Preparing for the Introduction of HPV Vaccine in the WHO European Region'. World Health Organisation <http://www.euro.who.int/__data/assets/pdf_file/0007/98746/E91432.pdf>

WHO (2009) 'Human Papillomavirus (HPV) Vaccine Background Paper'. September. Biotext Pty. Ltd., Canberra; <http://www.who.int/immunization/documents/HPVBGpaper_final_03_04_2009.pdf>

WHO (2016a) 'Vaccines.' World Health Organisation; <http://www.who.int/topics/vaccines/en/>

WHO (2016b) 'Human Papilloma Virus (HPV) and cervical cancer'. June; <http://www.who.int/mediacentre/factsheets/fs380/en/>

Wilyman, Judy (2011) 'Letter to 60 Minutes regarding the show 'Getting to the Point.' August 14; <http://sanevax.org/letter-to-60-minutes-regarding-the-show-getting-the-point/>

Wilyman, Judy (2015) 'A critical analysis of the Australian government's rationale for its vaccination policy'. Doctor of Philosophy Thesis. School of Humanities and Social Inquiry. University of Wollongong. 2015; <http://ro.uow.edu.au/theses/4541>

Wilyman, Judy (2016) 'Vaccination Decisions: Know Your Vaccines'; <http://vaccinationdecisions.net/about-us/>

Wright, T, F X Bosch, E L Franco, J Cuzick, J T Schiller, G P Garnett and A Meheus (2006) 'Chapter 30: HPV vaccines and screening in the prevention of cervical cancer; conclusions from a 2006 workshop of international experts'. Vaccine Supplement 24S3. June; <http://www.hu.ufsc.br/projeto_hpv/Chapter%2030%20HPV%20vaccines%20and%20screening%20in%20the%20prevention%20of%20cervical.pdf>

Yiwen, Cai (2016) 'China Approves First HPV Vaccine'. *Sixth Tone.* July 18; <http://www.sixthtone.com/news/china-approves-first-hpv-vaccine>

Zhao, Chengquan, Huaitao Yang and Zaibo Li (2014) 'Cytopathology and More Evidence Emerging for HPV-negative Cervical Cancer'. *Cap Today.* January; <http://www.captodayonline.com/cytopathology-and-more-evidence-emerging-for-hpv-negative-cervical-cancer/>

Zielinski, Alex (2016) 'After Japan Embraces 'Sensational' Anti-Vaxxer Report, HPV Vaccination Rates Collapse'. July 21; <https://thinkprogress.org/after-japan-embraces-sensational-anti-vaxxer-report-hpv-vaccination-rates-collapse-ab4a0c0505bb#.80enkf1qp>

If you would like to know more about Spinifex Press,
write to us for a free catalogue, visit our website
or email us for further information.

Spinifex Press
PO Box 105
Mission Beach QLD 4852
Australia

www.spinifexpress.com.au
women@spinifexpress.com.au